# Medical S Health Care Professionals

## A New Approach

Ronald W. Scott, PT, JD, EdD, MA (Spanish)
Attorney - Mediator
Clinical Physical Therapist - Educator
Cibolo, Texas

JONES AND BARTLETT PUBLISHERS
*Sudbury, Massachusetts*
BOSTON    TORONTO    LONDON    SINGAPORE

*World Headquarters*

Jones and Bartlett Publishers
40 Tall Pine Drive
Sudbury, MA 01776
978-443-5000
info@jbpub.com
www.jbpub.com

Jones and Bartlett Publishers
Canada
6339 Ormindale Way
Mississauga, Ontario L5V 1J2
Canada

Jones and Bartlett Publishers
International
Barb House, Barb Mews
London W6 7PA
United Kingdom

Jones and Bartlett's books and products are available through most bookstores and online book-sellers. To contact Jones and Bartlett Publishers directly, call 800-832-0034, fax 978-443-8000, or visit our website www.jbpub.com.

Substantial discounts on bulk quantities of Jones and Bartlett's publications are available to corporations, professional associations, and other qualified organizations. For details and specific discount information, contact the special sales department at Jones and Bartlett via the above contact information or send an email to specialsales@jbpub.com.

The authors, editor, and publisher have made every effort to provide accurate information. However, they are not responsible for errors, omissions, or for any outcomes related to the use of the contents of this book and take no responsibility for the use of the products and procedures described. Treatments and side effects described in this book may not be applicable to all people; likewise, some people may require a dose or experience a side effect that is not described herein. Drugs and medical devices are discussed that may have limited availability controlled by the Food and Drug Administration (FDA) for use only in a research study or clinical trial. Research, clinical practice, and government regulations often change the accepted standard in this field. When consideration is being given to use of any drug in the clinical setting, the health care provider or reader is responsible for determining FDA status of the drug, reading the package insert, and reviewing prescribing information for the most up-to-date recommendations on dose, precautions, and contraindications, and determining the appropriate usage for the product. This is especially important in the case of drugs that are new or seldom used.

**Library of Congress Cataloging-in-Publication Data**
Scott, Ronald W.
  Medical Spanish for health care professionals: a new approach/Ronald W. Scott.
    p. ; cm.
  Includes bibliographical references.
  English and Spanish.
  ISBN-13: 978-0-7637-4982-8
  ISBN-10: 0-7637-4982-6
  1. Spanish language–Conversation and phrase books (for medical personnel) I. Title.
  PC4120.M3S37 2008
  468.3'42102461–dc22
                          2007013276

6048
*Production Credits*
Executive Editor: David Cella
Editorial Assistant: Lisa Gordon
Production Director: Amy Rose
Production Editor: Renée Sekerak
Associate Marketing Manager: Jennifer Bengtson
**Printed in the United States of America**
11 10 09 08      10 9 8 7 6 5 4 3 2

Manufacturing and Inventory Coordinator: Amy Bacus
Cover Design: Kristin E. Ohlin
Composition: Pre-Press PMG
Printing and Binding: Malloy Incorporated
Cover Printing: Malloy Incorporated

# Contents

# Dedication

I dedicate this book with love to my wife Pepi. Thanks for your untiring support and love, and for your sage comments during your review of this book. I also dedicate the book to our two wonderful grandchildren, Isabel and Jonas.

# Prologue

You can do this! In fact, if you live and work almost anywhere in the United States, then you *must* learn at least elemental Spanish in order to communicate effectively with all of your patients. Currently, Hispanics with limited English proficiency (LEP) make up as much as 20 percent of the patient population in the United States. The ability to effectively communicate with these patients and their significant others is crucial for health care professionals' effective contributions to the health care delivery system and practice success.

I take a bold approach to learning what I call elemental Spanish—forget all (or most) the rules of grammar, linguistics, spelling and syntax. You are training to communicate with your Spanish-speaking patients—not to become a Spanish linguist.

This book presents a novel but simple approach to mastering elemental and basic conversational Spanish through incorporating a blend of English and Spanish. This dialect, commonly known as Spanglish, is frowned on by linguistic purists, but is the principal mode of communication between most English-speaking health care professionals and LEP patients and their significant others. Through early introduction of basic words and phrases through multiple drills and mastery of key health-related words, readers learn confidence in vital communications with their Spanish-speaking patients and clients. When you don't know certain words in Spanish in a sentence, try filling in the blanks with English. It is analogous to bricks and mortar. The theme throughout the book is "It really is as easy as it sounds!"

There are seven chapters in the book. Chapter 1, *Why Learn Spanish?*, addresses demographics, sociocultural considerations, and Spanish dialects throughout the world. Chapter 2, *You Are Not Trying to Become a Spanish Linguist*, looks at acceptable modes of interpersonal communication in general and the crucial nature of health care professional-patient communications in particular. The chapter also addresses the fundamentals of patient care documentation. Chapter 3, *You Already Know a Lot of Spanish*, includes a self-assessment quiz about how much basic Spanish one already knows and how to choose and use a Spanish-English dictionary in clinical practice. Chapter 4, *The Basics*, compares English and Spanish linguistics and phonetics, differentiates formalities and tenses in English and Spanish, explores comparative grammar and pronunciation, and provides basic communicative Spanish words and phrases. Chapter 5, *The Medical Nitty-Gritty—You Can Do This!*, covers clinical care activities such as patient intake, medical and social history taking, and the physical examination. Chapter 6, *Focus on Rehabilitation*, addresses focused topics like pain questions, special tests and measurements, gait analysis, therapeutic exercise, manual therapy techniques, and modalities. Chapter 7, *Special Considerations*, deals with translators, medical abbreviations, and techniques for effective communication with Hispanic patients and their significant others.

Features of each chapter include: bilingual vocabulary lists, practice drills, and patient-health care professional encounter scenarios. Each chapter is structured with a chapter abstract, multiple objectives, a summary, and end-of-chapter discussion questions. Three appendices include a quick guide made up of vital basic words and phrases for effective HCP-patient communications, and English-Spanish versions of a patient bill of rights and duties and a HIPAA privacy statement.

The book is intended for clinical health care professionals at all levels. The materials have been field-tested in a variety of clinical and in-service presentation scenarios.

Best wishes for continued practice success and service to patients!

# About the Author

Ron Scott, EdD, JD, MA, PT, is a certified bilingual primary and secondary teacher and university educator, a physical therapist, and an attorney-mediator. He divides his work time among these three disciplines. Ron began his health care career as a Navy hospital corpsman and operating room technician in 1970. He married his wife, Pepi, in her hometown of Puerto de Santa Maria, Spain, on August 5, 1973. Ron left military service initially in 1973 to study physical therapy at the University of Pittsburgh, where he was a student intern in the Center for International Studies. He has been a clinical physical therapist since 1977.

Ron attended law school at the University of San Diego from 1980 to 1983, where he was law review editor and symposium editor for the school's prestigious *Law of the Sea* issue. He subsequently served as an Army attorney-prosecutor and chief of international law in Frankfurt, Germany. After his return to the United States, Ron earned his postdoctoral Master of Laws degree from the JAG School, Charlottesville, Virginia, after which, he was an Army medical claims judge advocate until 1989.

Ron completed his 20-year military career as a physical therapist clinic director and senior staff member at Fort Polk, Louisiana and Brooke Army Medical Center, San Antonio, Texas. He had the opportunity to treat hundreds of Spanish-speaking patients in these and follow-on clinical settings. Ron retired as Major in 1994.

From 1994 to 1998, Ron was faculty and interim chair, Physical Therapy Department, the University of Texas Health Science Center, San Antonio, Texas. He coordinated two workshops in the Rio Grande Valley geared toward Hispanic health care professionals as part of an Area Health Education Center (AHEC) grant, and was featured in two health education presentations in Spanish on the local Univision television station.

Ron was a bilingual physical therapist at Corridor Medical Clinic, San Marcos, Texas, from 2002–2004, and bilingual physical therapist-in-charge at Health South-Crestway, from 2004–2005. He taught staff basic conversational Spanish, and interacted extensively with Spanish speaking patients and families.

Currently, Ron is adjunct faculty in four graduate health professional education programs—Husson College, Bangor, Maine; Marymount University, Arlington, Virginia; Rocky Mountain University, Provo, Utah; and the University of Indianapolis, Indianapolis, Indiana. Ron's current legal practice focuses on mediation and arbitration of interpersonal disputes.

Ron has published 11 other books, most recently *Guide for the New Health Care Professional,* Jones and Bartlett, 2007. He has also published over 60 articles, on topics ranging from cleidocranial dysplasia and snapping hip syndrome to health law and ethics to protecting United States interests in Antarctica.

Ron completed his Master of Arts, Spanish, with a concentration in linguistics, from Millersville University in 2003. He earned his Doctor of Education degree from the University of Texas at Austin in 2004.

*You only know as many people as you know languages.*
Napoleon Bonaparte

# Chapter 1

# Why Learn Spanish?

*One in seven United States citizens and residents is Spanish speaking. Spanish is an important world language. Only Chinese is spoken by more people. The United States is rapidly becoming a bilingual, or dual-language, nation. Bilingual education and English as a second language education programs are helping facilitate this transition. Spanish-language information permeates our everyday environment, making basic Spanish language accession more facile for everyone. Hispanic cultural development has played a key role in molding modern-day written and spoken Spanish. Although there are many dialects around the world, Latin-based Spanish is universally comprehensible to all.*

## OBJECTIVES

1. Appreciate that the Spanish language is the primary language of one in seven people in the United States.
2. Recognize why and how the United States is rapidly becoming a bilingual, or dual language, nation.
3. Examine the sociocultural aspects of the Spanish-speaking world.
4. Explore the various dialects of Spanish speakers.
5. Practice a basic exercise involving a Spanish-speaking patient and an English-speaking health care professional.
6. Fulfill fiduciary duties owed to patients under care, including the duty to impart fundamental care-related information and disclosure in patients' primary languages, with or without intermediaries.

1

## VOCABULARY

Andalucian Spanish

*Bajo latín* (common medieval Latin)

Bilingual education

*Bilingüe* (bilingual)

Castilian Spanish

*La chamaca, el chamaco* (girl, boy)[Mexico]

*La cita* (appointment)

*La clínica* (clinic)

*Coger* (to get or obtain) [Spain only]

*La comunicación* (communication)

*El consultorio pediatra particular* (pediatric private practice)

*El correo electrónico* (e-mail)

*Difícil* (difficult)

English as a second language (ESL)

English language learners

*Español* (Spanish)

*Fácil* (easy)

Fiduciary duty

*Hablar* (to talk)

*La/el hispanohablante* (Spanish-speaker)

Latin-American Spanish

Limited English proficiency

*Llamar* (to call)

*Lo siento* (I'm sorry)

*Mío* (mine)

*Nada* (nothing)

*La niña, el niño* (girl, boy)

Primary language

*Repetir* (to repeat)

Scaffolding

Secondary language

*Señor, Señora* (Mr., Mrs.)

Sheltered instruction

*Sí* (yes), *Si* (if)

Sociocultural theory

*Tener* (to have)

*La/el terapeuta ocupacional* (occupational therapist)

*La terapia* (therapy)

*El traductor, la traductora* (translator, male/female)

Transitional bilingual education

*Tú* (you, familiar, singular)

*Usted* (you, formal, singular)

*El volante* (referral order)

*Vos* (you, familiar, singular) [Argentina]

*Vosotros* (you, familiar, plural)

Zone of proximal development

# Demographics

As of July 1, 2006, there were 298,444,215 people living in the United States, according to the Central Intelligence Agency.[1] Of those, nearly

300 million people, some 40 million, are Spanish speakers (*hispanoh-ablantes*).[2]

The United States has the fifth-largest Spanish-speaking population in the world, behind Argentina, Columbia, Mexico, and Spain.[3] Some 400 million people around the world speak Spanish,[4] making it the second most-frequently spoken language on Earth, behind Chinese and ahead of English.[5]

Everyone everywhere has the basic human right to health care services, explained and delivered in languages that patients understand. Health care professionals in the United States must know enough elemental Spanish to communicate effectively with their Spanish-speaking patients in order to fulfill this duty owed to patients under their care.

*Health care professionals must be able to communicate effectively with all patients, with or without intermediaries, in order to fulfill the fiduciary duties they owe to patients under their care.*

# We Are a Bilingual Nation

Look around, and you will see evidence that the United States is a bilingual, or dual language, nation. What continues to make the United States such an attractive place to visit and live are the factors of choice, diversity, and freedom. Using the analogy of a food dish, the United States may not be a true melting pot, as it has been labeled so often in the past, but it is like a delicious rice bowl, adorned with a wide range of diverse condiments.

In San Antonio, Texas, where I live, Spanish is routinely spoken and seen everywhere—in movie theaters, outdoor advertising, restaurants, stores, and health care facilities. There are at least six Spanish-language television stations in the city and suburbs—including CNN-Español, Galavision, HBO-Latino, Telemundo, and Univision, which are watched by Spanish speakers and Spanish language learners alike. With near-constant audiovisual stimulation, the entire population of the area is slowly becoming elementally bilingual. The same situation exists in many urban areas in the United States, from Chicago to Miami to New York City to Phoenix to Salt Lake City. In these areas, and throughout the nation, Spanish-language information permeates the environment, making basic Spanish language accession more facile (easily attainable).

Canada represents the most classic example of a well-working dual-language nation. French has been an official Canadian language since 1968. The French language is predominant in Quebec Province, and is regularly spoken in other mostly eastern provinces, including New Brunswick, the only official bilingual province in Canada. Other languages spoken by Canadians, including Gaelic, have also enjoyed what are called "minority language educational rights" under the Canadian Constitution since 1982.[6]

There are several French-speaking enclaves in the United States, as well. Two of them are along the Maine-Canadian and Michigan-Canadian borders. Another is Louisiana, where French-Acadian (Cajun) immigrants settled in the 1700s.

Spanish is spoken nearly universally by 40 million people across the United States. Because of extensive internal migration of Spanish-speaking American citizens and residents, Spanish-speaking clubs, media, restaurants, schools, and other venues can be seen at all corners of the lower 48 and everywhere in between.

The United States' territory of Puerto Rico in the Caribbean Sea is a great example of a primary Spanish-speaking society within the United States. English and Spanish are both primary languages in Puerto Rico. While the vast majority of the population (3.8 million) list Spanish as their primary language, most Puerto Ricans in urban areas speak fluent English. However, primary-, secondary-, and post-secondary education in Puerto Rico is conducted in Spanish.

Bilingual education is both extensive and politically controversial in the United States. English language learners with limited English proficiency are given the opportunity to acquire English language competency over time. The most common type of bilingual education is transitional bilingual education, in which children learn academic subjects in a primary language other than English for up to three years while they incrementally acquire English language proficiency. The goal of this type of sheltered instruction is to mainstream students in the programs to English-only instruction as soon as possible. The autonomous English speaker is theoretically and practically developed through scaffolding, or temporary support—by teachers, fellow students, and families—along the way. According to education consultant Kathleen Kenfield, sheltered instruction is optimally useful for intermediate-level English language learners.[7]

Another type of bilingual education is late-exit or developmental bilingual education. In this mode, learners with limited English proficiency continue to receive academic education in their primary language, and progressively in English, for extended periods of time (beyond three years).

Still another model of bilingual education is dual language or two-way bilingual/biliterate education, in which English-speaking students interact on an ongoing basis with non-English-speaking classmates. Through this interaction and bilingual teaching/learning, all students learn English and a minority language simultaneously. This is considered highly effective for optimizing learning and long-term performance of English language learners.[8]

Bilingual education is common around the world, not just in the United States and Canada. One prominent example is the plurilingualism promotion plan that showcases bilingual education in the province of Andalucia in southern Spain. English, French, and German have been taught in 400 dual-language, bilingual school programs since 1998 as part of the province's initiative. (To see a complete copy of Andalucia's plurilingualism promotion plan, do a search on that phrase at www.wikipedia.org.[9])

English as a Second Language, or ESL, is a teaching/learning method that supplements or follows sheltered bilingual content education. It consists of daily subject-specific speaking, reading, and writing drills intended to improve the skills of English language learners. ESL is classified by proficiency level (e.g., beginner, intermediate, and advanced), rather than by grade level.

The antithesis of bilingual education or learning is immersion language learning. Immersion learning is "cold turkey" exposure to a new language. For immigrants—and especially for their children in public schools—this method can be a frightening and unjust way to acclimate them to English.

# Sociocultural Considerations

This section presents two levels of sociocultural considerations. The first level addresses sociocultural theory. The second focuses on sociocultural aspects of Hispanic people around the world.

Sociocultural theory, according to Vygotsky, holds that learning is embedded in social events. An individual's development of higher order thinking and functioning directly correlates with that individual's social interactions with other people, objects, and events in his or her environment. Social interactions are primarily cultural in nature. Infants and toddlers learn principally from their family members and caregivers. Young people are cultural apprentices who learn and develop from interactions with family, teachers and other authority figures, and peers. Everyone—including Spanish language learners like you—learns, is supported or scaffolded, and develops within a zone of proximal development.[10]

Culture refers to the beliefs, folklore, history, language(s), mores, norms, practices, and values of a defined social group and of individuals within that group.[11] Hispanic culture has two co-primary influences—Spain and its people, and Latin America and its indigenous societies. The cultural presentation of Hispanics around the world is a composite of their influences.

The culture of Spain has been heavily influenced by the Romans, Visigoths, and Moors who conquered, dominated, and shaped it, and by the Catholic reconquerors and Hebraic scholars (and their wives and significant others) who sustained it during those periods. Spain, or Hispania, at the southwestern edge of the Roman empire, was a center of commerce and culture. Seneca, the Roman dramatist, philosopher, and statesman, was born in Cordoba.[12]

The Visigoths invaded and took control of Spain in 414, ushering in the Middle Ages.[13] The Moors wrested control from the Visigoths in 711; renamed the caliphate *Al-Andalus,* and held the country until the last city, Granada, was recaptured in 1492, and the Catholic monarchs, Isabel and Ferdinand, expelled them (along with Spain's Jews).[14] The Arabs and Jews left Spain a framework for further development, including brilliant advances in architecture, literature, mathematics, and philosophy.

Spain sustained a Golden Age from approximately 1550 to 1650, in which it was the dominant world power. It led the world in art, commerce, drama, law, and politics. Its principal novelist, Miguel de Cervantes Saavedra (1547–1616), wrote and published *Don Quijote* in two installments (1605 and 1616). More copies of *Don Quijote* have been sold than any other book except the Bible and the Koran.

Spain went on to conquer most of the New World (North, Central, and South America). Its goals were to convert native populations to Christianity and to make Spain rich through mineral and other natural resources. In the process, many native cultures disappeared. Others melded into the existing milieu.

As happens with all world powers, competition, complacency, military defeats, and a series of unfortunate events led to the diminution of Spain's power. Spain lost most of its colonies through revolution. Simón Bolívar became the great liberator of South American countries, including Bolivia, Columbia, Equador, Panama, Peru, and Venezuela.[15]

Two devastating wars sealed Spain's fate as a defeated world power. In the Spanish-American War between Spain and the United States (1898), Spain lost most of its remaining colonies, including Cuba, Guam, Puerto Rico, and the Philippines. A national melancholy ensued, from which the great Spanish writers, called the Generation of '98, emerged—among them, Azorín, Baroja, Jiménez, Machado, and Unamuno.[16]

The Spanish Civil War raged from 1936–1939.[17] During that battle of ideologies between right and left, in which my father-in-law was a combatant, 1,000,000 Spanish died, and a fascist dictatorship, led by Francisco Franco, put a stranglehold on the "restoration" of Spain that the Generation of '98 had envisioned. Franco died in 1975; democracy returned, and Spain regained much of its world influence and mystique.

# Spanish Dialects Throughout the World

As the second most-spoken language on Earth, Spanish is relatively easy to learn and to listen to. Like French, Italian, Portuguese, and Romanian, Spanish is a Latin-based romance language. In the western Roman Empire (including Hispania), *bajo latín* (vulgar Latin)[18] was spoken instead of the classic Latin of Caesar and Cicero.

By the time an autonomous Spain was firmly established, five distinct languages were in place: Castilian (modern-day Spanish), spoken by the majority; Catalan, spoken in Barcelona and throughout the province of Catalonia; Basque, spoken in Bilbao and throughout the Basque country; Galician, a derivative language of Celtic-influenced Galician-Portuguese, spoken in northwestern Spain; and Romani, spoken by Spain's nearly one million gypsies.[19]

Spanish peninsular dialects carry minor differences. Castilian Spanish, spoken in Madrid, pronounces the letter "z" as "th." As a result, Castilians pronounce the city name Zaragoza as "Tharagotha." Andalucian Spanish also has interesting distinct colloquial variants, as do the dialects of the other 14 autonomous provinces of Spain.[20]

Latin American Spanish has co-opted the flavor of indigenous societies and of English. Latin Americans are more likely to use the term "e-mail," rather than the pure Spanish phrase *correo electrónico* used in Spain. Most of the world's Spanish speakers—300,000 of 400,000 people—live in Latin America and the United States.

Latin American dialects include, among others, Argentine, Caribbean, Cuban, Mexican, and Puerto Rican. Argentines use *vos* instead of *tú* for the singular version of you (familiar). Inhabitants of Buenos Aires speak with Neapolitan Italian accents. Mexican Spanish is infused with Nahuatl (Aztec) words, like *chamaco,* for *niño* (boy). Spoken Puerto Rican Spanish often displays a subtle blend of r's and l's, as in *Puelto Rico* and *Señol* (for *Señor,* Mr.). Throughout Latin America, grammatical use of *vosotros,* the complex informal "you" plural verb form is avoided.

The beauty of spoken and written Spanish is that it is fungible throughout the world, that is, all of its dialectal variants are readily understood by all. It is often said that among the many regional English accents found in the United States, Californians speak virtually without any accent. As a new elemental Spanish learner, you too should strive to speak without any particular accent.

When you are learning and using Spanish with patients, be careful to avoid using words and phrases that are unacceptable in specific regions. One prominent example is the Spanish verb *coger* (to get or obtain). The use of *coger* is indispensable in Spain, just as its English analog "to get" is in the United States. Yet in Latin America, it often carries the negative colloquial connotation "to fornicate."

---

*The beauty of spoken and written Spanish is that it is fungible throughout the world, that is, all of its dialectal variants are readily understood by all.*

---

Three excellent references on Spanish slang and sexually-oriented language are: D Burke, *Street Spanish 1 (Slang)* and *Street Spanish 3 (Naughty Spanish),* 1997, New York, John Wiley and Sons, and I Mendoza, *Hide This Spanish Book,* 2004, Singapore, Berlitz.

---

*When speaking Spanish with your patients, take care to avoid using words and phrases that may be unacceptable in specific regions. Example:* coger *("to get") [Spain], ("to fornicate") [Mexico].*

---

*Exercise #1: Read the following instructions. Translate the
English dialogue into Spanish to the best of your ability,
based on what you might say to the person at the other end
of the telephone connection.*

Background:
You are an occupational therapist (*terapeuta ocupacional*) in a pediatric private practice (*consultorio pediatra particular*). [Notice how the word order for words and phrases is sometimes reversed in Spanish, compared to English.] A patient named *Señora* (Mrs.) *Velázquez* calls for an appointment for her daughter *Ángela*.

Dialogue:
[Ring]

| | |
|---|---|
| OT: | ABC Pediatric Clinic. How may I help you? |
| Sra. Velázquez: | *Buenos días. Tengo un volante para mi hija Ángela, para una cita con su clínica.* |
| OT: | Hello? [Realizing that the person on the other end of the line may be speaking in Spanish] [Slowly] I'm sorry. I don't speak Spanish. Do you speak English? |
| Sra. Velázquez: | *No, lo siento, no hablo inglés.* |
| OT: | [Quickly fumbling for the key phrase—"telephone number"—in a Spanish dictionary.] *Número de teléfono?* |
| Sra. Velázquez: | *El mío? Dos-cero-uno-cinco-cinco-cinco-uno-nueve-ocho-cinco.* |
| OT: | I'm sorry, I didn't get that. Could you repeat it, please? Repeat-o? |
| Sra. Velázquez: | *Repítalo?* [Slowly] *Dos-cero-uno-cinco-cinco-cinco-uno-nueve-ocho-cinco.* |
| OT: | [Trying to spell out the number phonetically] *Dos-cero-uno-cinco-cinco-cinco-uno-nueve-ocho-cinco?* |
| Sra. Velázquez: | Sí. |
| OT: | [From the bilingual dictionary again, using the key phrase "May I call you back?" within the dictionary term "call back,"] *¿Puedo llamarte más tarde?"* |
| Sra. Velázquez: | Sí, por favor. |

[End conversation.]

Discussion: You don't understand much Spanish at this point, so there is little you can say in response to Sra. Velázquez's request for an appointment for her daughter Ángela. You were able to bridge with your Spanish dictionary. You need a Spanish-speaking receptionist or other staff member in your practice at this point, to take calls from Spanish-speaking clients, and to translate for you during patient care activities.

As a practical matter, are you going to be equally understood by Spanish-speaking patients if you inadvertently identify yourself using the incorrect word *terapista* instead of *terapeuta*? Yes. The goal of interpersonal communication at this elemental level is simply to be understood.

## SUMMARY

Learning elemental Spanish is relatively easy, and necessary in a modern-day medical or health professional practice. One in seven of your potential clientele is Spanish speaking. Augmenting self-study to crash courses to formal language study, constant exposure to Spanish in everyday media promotes language acquisition. Hispanic history and culture gave and give rise to a dynamic Latin-based language that is predictable and easy to speak and write. Be careful in practice to avoid overfamiliarity with patients, and even the accidental use of prohibited or precautionary words such as *coger,* which means "to get" in Spain, but "to fornicate" in Mexico.

## DISCUSSION QUESTIONS

1. Is the United States truly a bilingual nation? Why or why not? If so, what are the consequences of that conclusion?
2. Should Spanish be made an official language of the United States, or of any particular states or regions? Why or why not?
3. How do you feel about the Pledge of Allegiance being recited, or the Star-Spangled Banner being sung, in Spanish?
4. Should workers be permitted by law to speak in their primary languages in the workplace? Why or why not? If so, what qualifiers, if any, should be placed on this practice?
5. What is your opinion of bilingual education in the United States?

# REFERENCES AND READINGS

1. www.cia.gov.
2. www.wikipedia.org [Spanish speakers].
3. Ibid.
4. www.spanish-school.com.
5. www2.ignatius.edu.
6. www.wikipedia.org [French Canadian].
7. Kenfield K. *Planning for success for your English learners.* 2006, Murphys, CA: Kenfield Publications.
8. Center for Applied Linguistics, 2005, University of California at Santa Cruz.
9. www.wikipedia.org [bilingual education].
10. Vygotsky L. *Thought and language.* 1986, Cambridge, MA: MIT Press.
11. *Webster's 9th new collegiate dictionary.* 1985, Springfield, MA: Merriam-Webster.
12. Giner G, Rios L. *Cumbres de la civilización española,* 3d ed. 1966, New York: Holt, Rinehart and Winston.
13. Ibid.
14. Collins R. *The Arab conquest of Spain, 710-797.* 1998, Malden, MA: Blackwell Publishers.
15. www.bolivarmo.com/history.htm.
16. www.britannica.com.
17. Thomas H. *The Spanish Civil War.* 1961, New York: Harper Colophone Books.
18. Sanchez-Romeralo A, Ibarra F. *Antología de autores españoles antiguos y modernos.* 1972, Englewood Cliffs, NJ: Prentice-Hall, Inc.
19. Bercovici K. *Gypsies: Their life, lore, and legends.* 1983, New York: Greenwich House.
20. Teschner R. *Camino oral: Fonética, fonología y práctica de los sonidos del español.* 2000, New York: McGraw Hill Higher Education.

# Chapter 2

# You Are Not Trying to Become a Spanish Linguist!

*The purpose of this book is to help you communicate with Spanish-speaking patients and their significant others at the most elemental level. It is a first step in what hopefully will be a lifelong journey of second language, or what is called "L2" development. Effective communication—between health care providers and patients, and between and among health care team members—is crucial to successful patient care outcomes. Before carrying out examinations and rendering treatment, primary health care providers must give patients vital information about their care and receive informed consent. Often, a patient speaks Spanish (or some other language), and translator assistance is required. Patient care documentation is as important as the rendition of care itself. In many bilingual areas, patient documents are written in both English and Spanish to facilitate patient and provider understanding and communication.*

## OBJECTIVES

1. Recognize the importance of interpersonal communication, especially between health care professional and patient.
2. Utilize translators, whenever necessary, to ensure that Spanish-speaking patients and their significant others understand provider communications.
3. Develop a personal framework for imparting disclosure information to, and obtaining informed consent from, patients under your care.

4. Analyze patient care documentation systems in your practice, and adapt them for current and future Spanish-speaking patients and providers.

5. Practice using a Spanish-English dictionary to access key medical words and phrases to communicate with Spanish-speaking patients.

## VOCABULARY

*El acceso directo* (direct access)

*Ambulatorio* (ambulatory, outpatient)

*La atención al paciente* (patient care)

*La atención quirúrgica* (perioperative care)

*Los beneficios* (benefits)

*La carta* (letter)

*El consentimiento informado* (informed consent)

*La/el dentista* (dentist)

*El derrame cerebral* (cerebrovascular accident)

*El diagnóstico* (diagnosis)

*La dislocación* (dislocation)

*La documentación* (documentation)

*La enfermera, el enfermero* (nurse, female/male)

*Enfermo/a,* (sick)

*La enferma, el enfermo* (patient, female/male)

*El equipo de rehabilitación* (rehabilitation team)

*El equipo quirúrgico* (surgical team)

*El historial médico* (health record)

*La investigación* (research study)

*El médico, la médica* (doctor, male/female)

*Las metas* (goals)

*La negación informada* (informed refusal)

*La/el paciente* (patient)

*El paciente hospitalizado* (inpatient)

*La/el participante* (research subject)

*El problema* (problem)

*El pronóstico* (prognosis)

*Los riesgos importantes* (material risks)

*El seguro médico* (medical insurance)

*El sustituto* (surrogate decision maker)

*La/el terapeuta* (therapist)

*Los tratamientos alternativos* (alternative treatments)

# Health Care Professional-Patient Communication Is What Is Key

Effective communication—between health care professionals and patients (*los enfermos*) and relevant others—is crucial to successful patient care (*atención al paciente*) outcomes. To get your point across, you must be understood by the target listener. That truism is made even more important by the fact that ineffective communication to and about patients to others having an immediate need to know may result in health care malpractice liability for professional negligence.[1]

Professional negligence occurs whenever a clinical health care professional's conduct (action or failure to act, when required to do so) falls below minimally acceptable practice standards. Ineffective communication to patients, and about patients to other relevant health care providers, is a form of professional negligence.

*Ineffective communication to patients, and about patients to other relevant health care providers, is a form of professional negligence.*

Effective communication between health care providers and patients and their surrogate decision makers (*sustitutos*) and significant others entails imparting vital care-related information that is accurate, comprehensive, timely, and understood. This is true in acute care, cancer and cardiac care, geriatrics and pediatrics, and particularly in perioperative care (*atención quirúrgica*). The failure on the part of health professionals and patients to understand each other can mean the difference between life and death for patients.

*Effective communication between health care providers and patients entails imparting vital care-related information that is accurate, comprehensive, timely, and understood.*

Part of the obligation to communicate effectively with patients involves avoiding excessive medical jargon when explaining their conditions or procedures to them. Most patients have not attended health professional education programs, and do not understand technical medical language. It is like a foreign language to them. Confusing medical jargon is especially frightening to them while they are sick or injured, and in pain. Translate medical terms into lay terms, and communicate with patients at their level of comprehension—whether that is at the doctoral or sixth-grade level.

---

*As a healthcare professional, always translate medical terms into lay terms for patients and their significant others, and take care to communicate with them at their level of comprehension.*

---

Informed consent (*consentimiento informado*) is a key component of communication between primary health care professional and patient. Many state practice acts and professional association codes of ethics spell out in varying detail the precise information that must be imparted to patients under care. This section describes the general nature of informed disclosure and consent.

The following elements normally must be disclosed to the patient before examination or intervention. Patient (or surrogate) questions must be actively solicited and satisfactorily answered by a primary health care provider in order to meet the legal requirements for patient informed consent. The exact requirements for informed consent vary from state to state, however. The list that follows does not necessarily represent the law of any particular state. (See your facility or personal attorney for specific advice.)

Patient informed consent to examination involves disclosure and discussion of the patient's medical or other relevant diagnosis and the parameters of the intended examination. For a patient's consent to health care intervention to be legally sufficient, or "informed," the primary health care provider must relate the following elements to the patient in layperson's language at the level of patient understanding:

1. A description of the patient's health problem (*problema*), diagnosis (*diagnóstico*), and evaluative findings, and of the recommended intervention (*tratamiento médico*).

2. The material risks (*riesgos importantes*), if any, associated with the recommended intervention. Material risks include important "decisional" risks (including foreseeable complications associated with the recommended intervention) or precautions that would cause an ordinary, reasonable patient to think carefully when deciding whether to undergo or reject the recommended intervention.

3. The reasonable alternatives (*tratamientos alternativos*), if any, to the proposed intervention (i.e., other effective potential interventions that would be acceptable substitutes under legal standards of practice). The provider must be sure to include discussion of the relative risks and benefits of alternative interventions.

4. The expected benefits (*beneficios*), goals (*metas*), and prognosis (*pronóstico*) associated with the recommended intervention.

Providers should memorize the above elements and routinely cover each of them with every patient. After the applicable disclosure elements are imparted to a patient, the health care provider must solicit patient questions and answer them to the patient's satisfaction before proceeding on to either examination or intervention. If, after disclosure of pertinent care-related information, a patient refuses examination and/or intervention, then the patient's informed refusal (*la negación informada*) should be carefully documented in the patient's record.

When the English language is not a patient's primary language (or that of the surrogate decision maker, for patients lacking mental capacity), the provider must either speak to the patient (or surrogate) in a language that is understood or use the services of an interpreter to ensure patient comprehension of the informed consent disclosure elements. Careful documentation is recommended whenever an interpreter is employed during these processes. An example of documenting the services of an interpreter during informed consent disclosure appears below.

---

*As primary health care providers, always bear in mind that any health-related intervention is only a recommended intervention (even if prescribed or ordered by a doctor or other health care professional), unless and until the patient with legal and mental capacity (or the patient's surrogate decision maker) agrees to it.*

---

Information is also required to be presented, in the case of a research study (*investigación*), in a language that the subject (*participante*) understands.[2] Prudent risk management and federal regulations also require that a research subject's informed consent be documented in writing.[3]

ABC General Hospital

Rehabilitation Center, Physical Therapy Section

May 23, 200X/1600


S: 42 y o female patient with a diagnosis of multiple sclerosis, wheelchair-bound, referred for "evaluation, facilitative range of motion, and progressive exercise and ambulation, to tolerance." Patient is Spanish-speaking; Mrs. Gonzáles, Red Cross volunteer, acted as interpreter.

0: ...(Objective information)

A: ...(Assessment)

P: Begin active assistive range of motion today; standing at parallel bars, to tolerance. I obtained informed consent from the patient in Spanish through Mrs. Gonzáles, interpreter. Pt. verbalizes understanding of her diagnosis and my examination findings: the recommended intervention as outlined in Dr. Doe's order; the risks of muscle soreness, fatigue, and the slight risk of joint dislocation (*dislocación*) associated with exercise; and information about the alternative options of bed rest and limited activity in her wheelchair. I asked for her questions through Mrs. Gonzáles. She wanted to know how long sessions lasted. I told her 45 minutes to 1 hour each, but only to her tolerance. She verbalized satisfaction with the program as outlined and agreed to try it.

G: ...(Goals)

Reggie Hausenfus, PT, #07165733

Figure 2.1   *Example of Informed Consent Documentation Involving an Interpreter for the Patient*

- Examination and evaluative findings; diagnosis (or diagnoses)
- Description of the recommended intervention(s)
- Material (decisional) risks of possible harm or foreseeable complications associated with the recommended intervention(s)
- Expected benefits (goals) and prognosis
- Reasonable alternatives to the recommended intervention, including relative risks, benefits, and prognosis associated with reasonable alternative interventions (or no intervention)
- Solicit and satisfactorily answer patient questions

Figure 2.2    *Checklist Disclosure Elements for Patient Informed Consent to Intervention*

*Patients and research subjects (or their surrogate decision makers) have the right to have relevant health-related information presented to them in languages that they understand, so they can make informed decisions about whether or not to accept recommended care, or to participate in research studies, as appropriate.*

Communication in health care involves more than just communication with patients and their families and significant others. It also involves constant communication with other members of the health care delivery team. A team may be a surgical team (*equipo quirúrgico*) or rehabilitation team (*equipo de rehabilitación*), consisting of doctors (*médicos*), nurses (*enfermeras* [female], *enfermeros* [male]), therapists (*terapeutas*), and many other team members.

Delayed communication of vital patient data to other health care professionals (HCPs) having an immediate need to know is a form of professional negligence, or substandard care. So is the communication to other team members of patient information that is inaccurate or even imprecise. If a patient is injured as a result of such substandard care practices, health care malpractice liability and all of its adverse consequences may ensue.

How is communication about patients between and among health care professionals accomplished? Often it is accomplished through first-person communication in person (*en persona*) or by letter (*carta*).

Most of the time, however, routine patient information is communicated among health care providers co-treating that patient through patient care documentation (*documentación*), which is stored in the patient's health record (*el historial médico*).

## Documentation: The Key to Effective Communication

As part of the legal duty owed to patients, every primary health care provider is required by legal, professional, and business ethical standards to record clinically pertinent history, examination, evaluative, and intervention-related information about their patients and to maintain that information in the form of patient treatment records. Besides primary health care providers (i.e., those licensed independent practitioners who can legally interact with patients without the requirement of a prior examination and referral by another health care provider), other health care professionals interacting with patients in supportive or consultative roles have the same duty to record patient information (if they are privileged under law and by their organizations to document) and ensure that it is safeguarded.

It is a truism that patient care documentation must be patient-focused. In many bilingual areas, patient documents are written in both English and Spanish to facilitate patient and provider understanding and communication.

Providers must use people-first, active-voice language when describing patients, both orally and in writing. Mrs. Jones, for example, is "a 52-year-old woman presenting with right cerebrovascular accident (*derrame cerebral*)", not "a hemi."

Who can legally document information in patient records is a matter of federal and state law, organizational or systems policy, and customary practice. For inpatient records, therapeutic orders are normally written by physicians and surgeons attending individual patients. In most cases, no one except a physician can record information in the "Physician's Orders" section of an inpatient record, except where so permitted by law and custom, such as when a dentist (*dentista*) writes relevant orders for care for a specific patient. In outpatient patient care settings, however, especially in clinical settings in which no physician may be present, intervention orders are routinely written by primary health care providers other than physicians, for example, by physical therapists in direct access (*acceso directo*), or practice-without-referral, jurisdictions.

Patient care records take many forms. Two primary classifications of patient care records include inpatient (*paciente hospitalizado*) records and ambulatory (*ambulatorio*), or outpatient, records. (Some authorities consider emergency treatment records as a separate category of patient care records.) While in the past, original patient treatment records were required by law to be handwritten in all jurisdictions, modernly, both inpatient and ambulatory records may now be created originally and maintained, either in whole or in part, on a computer.

It is difficult to enunciate a precise definition for a patient care record. In simplest terms, a patient care record is a memorialization of a specific patient's health status at a given point in time. The patient treatment record includes clinically pertinent information that is clear, concise, comprehensive, individualized, accurate, objective, and timely. It serves both as a business document and as the legal record of care rendered to the patient.

From business and clinical perspectives, as well as from a legal standpoint, documentation of patient care is as important as the rendition of care itself. This axiom holds true for the protection of patients and health care professionals alike. For health care providers, patient care documentation is substantive evidence of the nature, extent, and quality of care rendered to patients, while for patients, it serves as a permanent record of their health status, which may, among many other purposes, serve as a historical record for future lifesaving intervention.

---

*Documentation of patient care is as important as the rendition of care itself.*

---

## Purposes of Patient Care Documentation

The patient care record serves a myriad of important purposes. Primary health care professionals and health care organizations act as fiduciaries, or persons and entities in a special position of trust *vis-à-vis* patients under their care. Therefore, logically, the primary purpose of patient care documentation is to communicate vital information about a patient's health status to other health care providers concurrently caring for that patient and having an imminent need to know the information contained therein. This principle operates either in an inpatient or outpatient care setting. The clinical information entered by one health care professional into a patient's record is assimilated by other providers into their intervention plans, and incorporated with their goals for patients—to ease discomfort, speed recovery, and maximize function and independence.

Despite what may be suspected by some to be the primary purpose for patient care documentation—self-protection from patient-initiated claims and litigation—this is clearly not the case. That kind of negative approach to documentation serves no positive purpose and only instills fear in health care professionals. Such fear, in turn, fosters an atmosphere of costly defensive health care practice.

A defensive posture regarding patient care documentation may actually increase the chances of malpractice exposure. Patients and their significant others can readily sense a health care provider's defensiveness. They justifiably find distasteful the kind of formal, cold, business-like relationship that inherently results when a health care professional puts fear of malpractice exposure (or other self-interest, such as revenue maximization) ahead of the patient's welfare. If patients come to believe that their health care providers are excessively focused on self-protection from litigation exposure or other selfish considerations, then they may be more inclined to pursue legal actions if and when an adverse outcome results from intervention.

There are many other important purposes for patient care documentation. Documentation of patient care serves as a basis for planning and for ensuring continuity of care in the future for patients currently under care, particularly for those inpatients who, after discharge, will require health professional intervention at home. By memorializing a patient's health status at any given point, documentation also serves to create a historical record of a given patient's health, from which data can be extracted for and utilized in future contingencies, ranging from emergent life-threatening crises to disability determinations.

Documentation also forms the basis for monitoring and assessing the quality of care rendered to patients as part of a quality management program. Such programs are required of health care facilities accredited by entities such as the Joint Commission on the Accreditation of Healthcare Organizations ("Joint Commission"), the Commission on Accreditation of Rehabilitation Facilities (CARF), the National Committee on Quality Assurance (NCQA), and others, including local, state, and federal public oversight entities.

Besides its utility as a database for monitoring and evaluating the quality of patient care, patient care documentation is useful as a productivity measure of provider workloads, and to assess whether health care providers are practicing effective utilization management of human and nonhuman health care resources. It also serves, through identifying deficiencies, to ascertain whether there are needs for training for health care providers, from communication skills to substantive aspects of patient care.

As a business document, the patient care record is also evaluated by governmental third-party payer entities such as Medicare, Medicaid, TRICARE (for military beneficiaries), and state and local governmental entities, and by medical insurance (*seguro médico*) companies and other third-party payers to determine levels of reimbursement for patient care. Documentation of patient care, then, is the primary means of justifying reimbursement for treatment. The treatment record also provides information that is useful for scientific and clinical research and for education.

Besides being a business document, the patient care record is a legal document as well. In the event of a health care malpractice claim or lawsuit, providers' documentation of patient care activities provides substantive and relatively objective evidence of the care that was rendered to the patient claiming malpractice. Documented evidence of care recorded in the patient's record provides expert witnesses with a basis from which to form a professional opinion on whether a provider or multiple providers met or violated standards of practice and legal standards of care. Patient care documentation also serves many other legal functions, including, among others, its use as substantive evidence of work or functional capacity in workers' compensation and similar administrative proceedings.

As an additional legal issue, documentation of patient informed consent protects patients, providers, and health care organizations and systems by serving as written evidence that a patient actually understood the risks and benefits of specific interventions and made a knowing, informed choice to undergo examination and accept recommended interventions. Documentation of a patient's desires in the event of that patient's mental incapacitation through advance directives serves also to memorialize patient decisions, evidence respect for patient autonomy, and to protect health care professionals who must carry out the patient's valid advance directives.

## Purposes of Patient Care Documentation

1. Communicates vital information about a patient's health status to other health care providers concurrently caring for that patient and having an imminent need to know the information contained therein.

2. Acts as a basis for patient-care planning and continuity of care.

3. Serves as the primary source of information for assessing the quality of patient care rendered.

4. Provides information for reimbursement and utilization review decisions.

5. Identifies provider deficiencies and training needs.

6. Serves as a resource for research and education.

7. Serves as a business document.

8. Serves as a multi-purpose legal document.

9. Provides substantive evidence on whether providers' care—and health care organizations' oversight of patient care activities—met or violated legal standards of care.

10. Memorializes patient informed consent to examination and intervention, as well as patient desires regarding life-sustaining measures in the event of a patient's subsequent mental incapacitation, through advance directives.

---

*Exercise #2: Imagine that you are the physical therapist-in-charge of a small outpatient clinic. You are asked by the clinic director to develop a brief (75 words or less) informed consent checklist for crutch walking for patients. Your patient population includes a substantial number of Spanish-speaking clients. Use the chapter vocabulary, checklist disclosure elements for patient informed consent to intervention, and any Spanish-English dictionary to help you develop the Spanish version of your informed consent checklist. Assume, for purposes of this exercise, that the problem that warrants crutches is difficulty with walking; the benefits of crutches include mobility and weight-bearing ability; the main risk of using crutches is falling; reasonable alternatives to using crutches include using*

*a walker or wheelchair; and the prognosis for recovery for most*
*patients is excellent with crutches. If there are words that you*
*are uncomfortable trying to translate, write them out in*
*English, but try to make your sentences, phrases, and words*
*flow smoothly. Be sure to include the following Spanish*
*words in your work product:*

---

*Los beneficios* (benefits)

*El consentimiento informado*
(informed consent)

*El diagnóstico* (diagnosis)

*Las metas* (goals)

*El problema* (problem)

*El pronóstico* (prognosis)

*Los riesgos importantes* (material
risks)

*La/el terapeuta* (therapist)

*Los tratamientos alternativos*
(alternative treatments)


The Spanish phrase for "crutch walking" is *andar con muletas.* Good
luck!

## SUMMARY

Effective patient-health care provider communications are so important that they often mean life or death for patients. Failure to communicate effectively with patients and their significant others constitutes
professional negligence, a form of health care malpractice. In a rapidly
growing Hispanic world, health care professionals at all levels in the
United States must be or become at least elemental in speaking Spanish in order to reach these patients and clients.

Similarly, interpersonal communications between and among health
care team members co-treating patients is crucial for successful patient
care outcomes. Patient care documentation must be accurate, concise,
legible, relevant, and timely. Computerized documentation systems
may aid in translation from English to Spanish and vice versa.[5]

Patient informed consent documentation and oral communications must also serve Spanish-speaking patients and their surrogate
decision makers. This chapter presents basic Spanish-language
informed-consent vocabulary, as well as a rudimentary exercise in
its utilization.

## DISCUSSION QUESTIONS

1. Linguists have concluded that learning each successive language beyond L2 becomes easier and easier. Do you agree? Why or why not? Does it matter that L3 (Arabic, for example) is not Latin-based, if L2 (Spanish, for example) is?

2. What steps can you take personally to facilitate and improve communications with existing and future Spanish-speaking patients in your practice?

3. Does your facility have a Spanish-language informed consent policy statement? If not, what steps can you take to help create one? Is there also a need to publish such a policy statement in other languages?

4. Does your practice or facility have dual-language patient care documentation forms? Are they necessary? If so, how can you initiate the process for their creation and implementation?

## REFERENCES AND READINGS

1. Scott R. Legal aspects of documenting patient care for rehabilitation professionals, 3rd ed. 2006, Sudbury, MA: Jones and Bartlett.
2. See 45 Code of Federal Regulations 46.116.
3. See 45 Code of Federal Regulations 46.117.
4. Halperin J, Healey J, Zeitchik E, Ludman W, Weinstein L. Developmental aspects of linguistic and mnestic abilities in normal children. J Clin Exp Neuropsychol. 1989; 11(4): 518–528.
5. Hutchins J. Twenty years of translating and the computer. ASLIB Conference, London, Nov. 13–14, 1998.
6. Halperin J. et al.

# Chapter 3

# Starting Up

*Second language acquisition occurs in much the same way as primary language acquisition—gradually, incrementally, and within a supportive communicative environment. Some English speakers need to become elementally conversant with Spanish speakers relatively quickly. This is the case with English-speaking clinical health care professionals practicing in an environment where there are Spanish-speaking patients. "Spanglish" is an acceptable early means to communicate with patients, and an effective adjunct to scaffolding to advanced Spanish language learning. All modern languages co-opt words and phrases from other languages. English is no exception. You may already know at least 100 to 150 Spanish words from everyday life. As you study and learn Spanish, facilitate your progress with a comprehensive general Spanish-English dictionary.*

## OBJECTIVES

1. Begin to develop self-confidence as you embark on early acquisition learning of elemental Spanish.
2. Create and practice using 3 x 5″ vocabulary cards to master medical Spanish words you have encountered in this book and elsewhere.
3. Recognize the potential value of Spanglish in early Spanish language acquisition.

4. Reflect upon and celebrate how much fundamental Spanish you already know by taking the self-assessment quiz at the end of the chapter.

5. Carefully evaluate, purchase, and use a comprehensive general Spanish-English dictionary.

## VOCABULARY

*El chequeo* (medical checkup)[Spanglish]

*El final* (closure)

*La grocería* (grocery store)[Spanglish]

*Logear* (to log in)[Spanglish]

*El lonche* (lunch)[Spanglish]

Spanglish

*Vocabulario* (lexicon)

# You Are Striving to Become Conversational in Elemental Spanish

You were introduced to 30 Spanish words and phrases in Chapter 1, and to an additional 29 Spanish clinically-related words and phrases in Chapter 2. Many or most of these words and phrases should be useful to you in your practice. As you read the rest of this book and study beyond, begin to assimilate these words and the new ones introduced in this and subsequent chapters into your personal lexicon. Second language acquisition begins with the first few words you understand, can put together, and use to communicate.

Consider creating and frequently reviewing a set of Spanish 3 x 5″ vocabulary flashcards. Don't worry about learning to write Spanish at this point. And don't worry too much about your pronunciation of Spanish words that you begin to use with patients and others. They will all be impressed because you are trying to converse with them in their primary language.

Every time I visit foreign countries, I try to assimilate a few dozen key words and phrases of the native languages into my working vocabulary. Be it Arabic, Czech, French, German, or Portuguese, I try to show that I am making an effort to communicate with locals in their language. In virtually every case, they express appreciation for the attempt, however rudimentary it may seem. Similarly, Spanish-speaking patients appreciate your efforts to converse with them in Spanish. It shows that you care and that you are serious about meeting the fiduciary duties that you owe them.

Always remember to keep your eyes on the prize—basic competency in elemental Spanish. Your goal in reading this book is to establish a foundation from which to build, so that you can converse with your patients and colleagues in Spanish at ever-improving levels of expertise.

---

*Spanish-speaking patients appreciate your efforts to converse with them in Spanish. It shows that you care and that you are serious about meeting the fiduciary duties you owe them.*

---

## How Do Language Learners with Limited Proficiency Communicate?

When you are attempting to learn a new language such as Spanish, reflect carefully on how you learned English as a child. Initial second language acquisition should be similar to first language acquisition— a gradual, low-pressure, supportive process in which errors are expected, tolerated and not emphasized by listeners.

Krashen calls this early, informal, subconscious second language learning "acquisition learning."[1] He labels later formal structured second language learning (as in a college course at night) as "the learning system." An effective filtering mechanism (in large part, self-perception) differentiates highly successful and less successful second language learners. Second language learners with high confidence, motivation, self-esteem, and support logically fare better in language acquisition than those at the opposite extreme.

So, chill out! Relax! Go slowly! Language competency is global, gradual, and multidimensional, rather than accomplished rapidly and along a straight-line continuum.[2] You will make many mistakes along the way. Don't strive early to be a perfectionist. Your patients will understand you and support you if you just try and persevere.

## Spanglish, Tex-Mex, and Derivatives Are Acceptable Modes of Interpersonal Communication

At this elemental level of Spanish language development, the use of customary colloquial Spanish—especially including Spanglish, Tex-Mex, and derivatives—are thoroughly acceptable. In fact, using Spanglish may be the only way early on that you can put sentences together coherently.

When I was a graduate student in Spanish at Millersville University in Pennsylvania, my advisor, mentor, and most respected professor, the late Dr. Rosario Caminero, a preeminent Spanish language linguist, always urged us to exercise caution regarding the use of Spanglish for Spanish language learners. I agree with Dr. Caminero's philosophy that, once students are beyond first-stage acquisition learning and in a formal, structured second language learning system, Spanglish is probably inappropriate for language learners, except in a cultural or dialectical context. For beginners, however, its use is invaluable.

In his book titled *Spanglish: The Making of a New American Language*,[3] Professor Ilan Stavans of Amherst College describes Spanglish as the key to the soul of a large portion of the Hispanic population—not just transitional English language learners, but also novelists and poets. Stavans' book presents and interprets hundreds of the current Spanglish words currently in use in the United States.

Think about how often Spanish-speaking patients and friends mix English and Spanish words and phrases as they converse and communicate with you and others. Words like *chequeo* for medical checkup, *grocería* for grocery store, *logear* for log in, and *lonche* for lunch are just a few examples of this phenomenon.

What then is Spanglish? Spanglish is the comingling and juxtaposition of Spanish and English words and phrases that are necessary or expedient and used principally by Spanish speakers to communicate with English speakers and others. There are as many different kinds of Spanglish as there are Hispanic ethnicities. Among Chicanos, Cubans, Dominicans, Ecuadorians, Mexicans, Puerto Ricans, Spanish, Tejanos, and others, Spanglish is a mixed, evolving language in significant use in the United States, Central and South America, and Spain.

For English speakers beginning to learn Spanish and needing an ability to converse right away, Spanglish can be a good early adjunct for scaffolding learning and communicating. This is especially true for health care professionals who need to communicate with their

Spanish-speaking patients. Spanglish should not be carried over, however, to advanced, formal, structured Spanish language learning.

---

*Spanglish: the comingling and juxtaposition of Spanish and English words and phrases; an evolving language in substantial use.*

---

# You Already Know a Lot of Spanish

Every modern language co-opts foreign words and phrases into its own language. Certain words—mostly colloquial in the case of American English—just don't translate well into other languages, and so are just adopted into everyday speech. For example, words and phrases like "bitchin'," "e-mail," and "rock and roll" are unique to American English. Similarly, French words like "champagne" and "reconnaissance" have become universalized. German words that are universally used include "bildungsroman," "gesellschaft," and "gestalt." Even extinct languages, like Virginia Algonquit, spoken by Pocahontas,[4] have contributed common words to the English lexicon, including "raccoon" and "moccasin."

Adolph Hitler tried unsuccessfully during the Third Reich to rid the German language of French and other foreign words. His efforts were futile, of course, because every modern language co-opts important useful words from other languages.

You might be surprised at how many Spanish words you already have in your working vocabulary. (The average adult in the United States has as many as 50,000 words in her or his working vocabulary.[5]) Take the self-assessment quiz below to see how many of the 257 words presented you already know and/or use, and can define.

---

*Every modern language co-opts important useful words from other languages.*

---

## Self-Assessment Quiz (English Words Co-opted or Derived from Spanish)

Put a check in front of the following Spanish words that you know and/or use in everyday speech. Many of these words are common restaurant food menu items. Can you think of any others? Add them at the end.

___Adiós

___Adobe

___Aficionado

___Alameda

___Alamo

___Albino

___Alcove

___Alfalfa

___Alligator

___Alpaca

___Amigo

___Aqua

___Armadillo

___Armada

___Arroyo

___Avocado

___Bachata

___Banana

___Bandoleer

___Barbeque

___Barracuda

___Barrio

___Bizarre

___Boca Raton [You know it's a city name, but what does it mean?]

___Bolas

___Bolero

___Bonanza

___Bonito

___Bronco

___Buckaroo

___Buenos días

___Buenas noches

___Burrito

___Burro

___Caballero

___Cabana

___Cacique

___Cafeteria

___Caldera

___Calor

___Camarilla

___Camino

___Canary

___Canasta

___Cannibal

___Canoe

___Canyon

___Caramba

___Caramel

___Carbonado

___Cargo

___Caribbean

___Carne

___Cha-cha

___Chaps

___Chicano

___Chica

___Chicle

___Chico

___Chihuahua

___Chili

___Chipotle

___Chocolate

___Chula Vista [Again, a city name, meaning what?]

___Churrasco

___Churro

___Cigar

___Cigarette

___Cilantro

___Cinch

___Coca

___Cocaine

___Coco

___Colorado

___Compadre

___Comprende

___Conquistador

___Condor

___Corral

___Coyote

___Creole

___Cumbia

___Demarcation

___Dengue

___Desaparecidos

___Desperado

___Dolor

___Don

___Dorado

___El Dorado

___El Niño

___Embarcadero

___Embargo

___Enchilada

___Espadrilles

___Fajitas

___Fandango

___Fiesta

___Filibuster

___Flamenco

___Flamingo

___Flan

___Flauta

___Fletcher

___Florida

___Flotilla

___Frijol

___Galleon

___Garbanzo

___Guacamole

___Gorro

___Guava

___Guerrilla

___Guitar

___Habanera

___Hacienda

___Hammock

___Hermosa

___Hermoso

___Hola

___Hombre

___Hoosegow

___Hurricane

___Inca

___Iguana

___Incommunicado

___Jaguar

___Jalapeño

___Jerky

___Junta

___Key

___La Niña

___Lariat

___Lasso

___Latino

___Linda

___Llama

___Lobo

___Loco

___Luminary

___Machete

___Machismo

___Macho

___Maize

___Majordomo

___Manatee

___Mantilla

___Mano

___Maquiladora

___Margarita

___Mariachi

___Marijuana

___Maroon

___Matador

___Merengue

___Mesa

___Mescal

___Menudo

___Mesquite

___Mestizo

___Mole

___Montana

___Mosquito

___Mulatto

___Mustang

___Nacho

___Nada

___Negro

___Nevada

___Nopal

___Olé

___Oregano

___Paella

___Palmetto

___Palomino

___Pampa

___Papaya

___Parasol

___Paso doble

___Patio

___Peccadillo

___Peon

___Peso

___Peyote

___Philippines

___Picaresque

___Pimento

___Piña colada

___Piñata

___Pinta

___Pinto

___Placer

___Plantain

___Platinum

___Playa

___Plaza

___Plume

___Poncho

___Posada

___Potato

___Pronto

___Pronunciamento

___Pueblo

___Puerto Rico

___Puma

___Quadroon

___Quesadilla

___Quirt

___Quixotic

___Ranch

___Reconquista

___Reefer

___Renegade

___Rodeo

___Rumba

___Salsa

___Samba

___Sarsaparilla

___Sassafras

___Suave

___Savanna

___Savvy

___Serape

___Serrano

___Shack

___Sherry

___Sierra

___Siesta

___Silo

___Sombrero

___Spaniel

___Spur

___Stampede

___Stevedore

___Stockade

___Tobacco

___Taco

___Tamale

___Tango

___Tapioca

___Tejano

___Tequila

___Tilde

___Tomatillo

___Tomato

___Torreador

___Tornado

___Tortilla

___Tuna

___Vamoose

___Vanilla

___Vaquero

___Vigilante

___Visa

___Yam

___Yerba mate

___Yucca

___Zorro

*Additional Spanish words co-opted into English?*

1. _____
2. _____
3. _____
4. _____
5. _____
6. _____
7. _____
8. _____
9. _____
10. _____

Scoring: Add up your total. Give yourself one point for each word you recognize and can define. Give yourself an additional two points for each additional Spanish word co-opted into English that does not appear on the list. Be sure to Google your additional words to ensure that they are actually Spanish derivative words (vs. French, Latin, etc.).

If you scored between 200–259+, your grade for the quiz is "A."
If you scored between 150–199, your grade for the quiz is "A-."
If you scored between 100–149, your grade for the quiz is "B."
If you scored between 50–99, your grade for the quiz is "B-."
If you scored less than 50, your grade for the quiz is C."

## Get and Use a Good Spanish-English Dictionary

You will recall that in Chapter 2, you used any Spanish-English dictionary to create a rudimentary informed consent checklist for patients requiring crutches. Evaluate this dictionary. Was it easy to use? Was it adequate in terms of containing the terminology that you sought?

I recommend that you purchase and use a comprehensive general Spanish-English dictionary. There are a myriad of good Spanish-English dictionaries in the marketplace, so carefully evaluate several before making your purchase decision, as they are expensive.

When you are evaluating Spanish-English dictionaries for purchase and use with patients, consider the following variables. The dictionary you select for purchase should include a substantial number of words and phrases in Spanish and English (in separate sections)—at least

250,000 words. It should include up-to-date colloquial and business words and phrases, as well as medical terminology. It should also include key phrases and useful sentences within word definitions. Your dictionary should be pre-tabbed for quick reference.

A comprehensive Spanish-English dictionary should also include a guide to the culture and dialects of the Spanish-speaking world, as well as a pronunciation guide. Your dictionary should optimally also include a correspondence guide, with formats for letter-writing in various settings, and Spanish verb tables.[6]

Once you have purchased and become familiar with your comprehensive Spanish-English dictionary, consider taking off the jacket cover. Your book should get a lot of use, and a floppy jacket cover will just impede your speed of access to vital words and phrases. Put it on your desk at work, and feel confident that you are rapidly learning and mastering elemental Spanish to better serve your patients.

---

*Exercise #3: Create and try to translate the following passage about directions to your clinic into Spanish/Spanglish. Use as many Spanish words and phrases as you know, and fill in the rest of the passage with Spanglish and/or English words and phrases. Make up details along the way to match your actual clinical setting, or invent a hypothetical clinical setting. Be sure to end the conversation with an appropriate closure or* final. *Relax, and good luck!*

---

[Phone rings]
       You:    ABC Medical Clinic. How may I help you?
Sra. Lopez:    Yes, *¿dónde,* um, where, *está* your *clínica, por favor?*
       You:    The *clínica? Sí,* it is ....

## SUMMARY

You have begun to learn the basic Spanish words and phrases that will be useful to you in your health care clinical practice. Spanglish can be a good early adjunct for scaffolding learning and communicating with Spanish-speaking patients, as long as it is not overused or carried over to formal, structured Spanish language learning.

Spanglish is the comingling and juxtaposition of Spanish and English words and phrases that are necessary or expedient and used principally by Spanish speakers to communicate with English speakers and others. There are as many different kinds of Spanglish as there are

Hispanic ethnicities. English speakers, too, can utilize Spanglish to communicate with Spanish speakers, such as patients under your care.

The number of Spanish words you already know because they have been co-opted into English probably exceeds 100. After purchasing a comprehensive Spanish-English dictionary, take time to ensure that you understand the meanings of the co-opted words that you recognize.

## DISCUSSION QUESTIONS AND ACTIVITIES

1. How comfortable do you feel speaking elemental Spanish? Are you surprised that so many Spanish words have been co-opted into the English lexicon?
2. What is your opinion on the value for Spanish language learners of watching Spanish language television, for example, news broadcasts such as CNN-Español?
3. What do you think about using Spanglish as an adjunct to scaffolding you to higher-level Spanish language learning? What are the risks of relying too heavily or too long on Spanglish to communicate with Spanish-speaking patients and others?
4. Select another major language like Chinese, French, or German, and come up with least 10 words from that language that have been co-opted into English.
5. Which Spanish-English dictionaries did you compare? Which one did you select, and why? After having used your dictionary for a month, are you still satisfied with your decision?

## REFERENCES AND READINGS

1. Krashen S. *Explorations in language acquisition and use*. 2003, Portsmouth, NH: Heinemann Publishers.
2. Ovando C, Collins V, Combs M. *Bilingual and ESL classrooms: Teaching in multicultural contexts*. 2005, New York: McGraw-Hill. HarperCollins Books.
3. Stavans I. *Spanglish: The Making of a New American Language*. 2003, New York: HarperCollins Books.
4. Wilford JN. Linguists find the words, and Pocahontas speaks again. *New York Times*. Mar. 7, 2006, F1.
5. Wren S. Developing research-based resources for the balance reading teacher. www.balancedreading.com [vocabulary].
6. Carvajal C, Horwood J, Jarman B, Russell R, eds. *The Oxford Spanish Dictionary*, 2nd ed., rev. 2001, New York: Oxford University Press.

# Chapter 4

# The Basics

*Spanish and English linguistics differ in many fundamental ways. Spanish is a Latin language; English is largely Germanic. Compared to English, Spanish vowel sounds are relatively simple to learn and use. What you see is literally what you get. While there are many more verb tenses in Spanish than in English, most conversations with patients take place in the simplest tense—the present indicative. This chapter introduces five basic verbs in the present indicative tense, and a wide array of key words and phrases for early mastery. Readers are urged to "fill in the gaps" of missing Spanish knowledge with English and/or Spanglish, to communicate better with Spanish-speaking patients under care. For critical conversations, however, translators may be required.*

## OBJECTIVES

1. Overview the differences between Spanish and English linguistics and phonetics.
2. Review basic Spanish and English rules of grammar.
3. Learn and use in practice five basic Spanish verbs in the present indicative tense.
4. Learn and use greetings, introductions, farewells, and other key Spanish words in practice.
5. Practice and master a basic introductory conversation between a health care provider and patient.

## VOCABULARY

Accentual rhythm

*El adjetivo* (adjective)

*El adverbio* (adverb)

*El agua* (water)

*El andador* (walker)

*El artículo* (article)

*La/el artista* (artist)

*El brazo, los brazos* (arm/arms)

*La casa* (house)

*Casada/o* (married)

Closed vowels

*La conferencia* (conference)
  [Also *el congreso*]

*Las conjunciones* (conjunctions)

*Determinado* (definite)

Diphthong

*El, la, las, lo, los* (the)

*El empleado, la empleada*
  (employee)

*El ejemplo* (example)

*Enfermo/enferma* (ill)

*La/el estadounidense* (American)

*Estar* (to be)

*Europeo/a* (European)

*Feliz* (happy)

Grammar

*Grande* (big)

Grapheme

*Hacer* (to do or make)

*Hay* (there is…)

*La hembra* (female)

*La hora* (hour, time)

*Indeterminado* (indefinite)

*Ir* (to go)

*El lápiz* (pencil)

*El libro* (book)

Linguistics

*Lunar* (surface of the moon; mole)

*El macho* (male)

*La/el modelo* (model)

Morphology

*La oficina* (office)

Open vowels

Orthography

*El papel* (paper)

*La perra, el perro*
  (female/male dog)

Phoneme

Phonetics

Phonics

*La pierna* (leg)

*La/el poeta* (poet)

*Por favor* (please)

*Por qué* (why)

*Porque* (because)

Predicate

*La preposición* (preposition)

*El pronombre* (pronoun)

*Rápidamente* (quickly)

Semantics

*Ser* (to be)

*El sustantivo* (noun)

Syllabic rhythm

Syntax

*Trabajar* (to work)

*Tener* (to have)

*Triste* (sad)

*Un, una* (a)

*Unos, unas* (some)

*El verbo* (verb)

*La vez* (time, as in *una vez,* "one time," or once)

# Comparative Spanish and English Linguistics and Phonetics

Linguistics is the study of language. There are two aspects to language study—its structure, or grammar, and its semantics, or meaning. Grammar is subdivided into two areas—morphology, or word makeup, and syntax, rules about the structure of sentences and phrases. Linguistics does not just include the study of spoken language, but also of language in its written form.

Phonetics is the study of human word sounds—how they are made and how they are understood by listeners. The smallest units of sound are called phonemes.

There are several fundamental linguistic differences between spoken and written Spanish and English. English is a Germanic language. Spanish is Latin-based. Spoken English is accentual in its rhythm; spoken Spanish is syllabic, i.e., the duration of enunciation of each syllable is identical. Spelling (orthography) in English is relatively difficult among world languages because words are spelled historically instead of phonologically. (The words "phone" and "thought" are examples of this phenomenon.) In Spanish, words generally sound exactly like they are spelled.

There are alphabetic differences between English and Spanish, too. The English alphabet contains 26 Latin letters (graphemes). Five of these letters (a, e, i, o, and u) are vowels, and the rest are consonants. The Spanish alphabet contains 29 letters, including all of the English/Latin graphemes, plus two digraphs (double letters with a single sound), "ch" and "ll," and the letter "ñ."

## Spanish Vowels and Vowel Sound Drills

Vowels are "open" letters compared to consonants, enunciated without constriction when the mouth and pharynx are open. They form the nucleus of syllables. One of the many pleasant aspects of learning Spanish vowel sounds is that they are relatively simple compared to English vowel sounds. Generally, what you see is what you get in terms of pronunciation. There are few surprises.

The five basic Spanish vowels sound like this:

1. "a"—like the English "a" in the words "ha, ha, ha"
2. "e"—like the English "a" in the month of "May"
3. "i"—like the English double "ee" in the word "meet"
4. "o"—just like our "o"
5. "u"—like the "u" in "lunar"

Try saying them in order, like you learned to recite the vowels in English as a child. Repeat them five times. Remember that every time you say them in spoken Spanish, or see them in written Spanish, this is how they will sound.

---

*Exercise #4: Repeat the sequence of Spanish vowel sounds daily until they are as familiar to you as English language vowel sounds. Remember them. They will be the foundation of your elemental conversational competence.*

---

You may still have a question about where, if anywhere, the English "i" vowel sound appears in the Spanish language. Two of the five vowel sounds in Spanish—"i" and "u"—are relatively closed compared with the other three, because mechanically the tongue is elevated when enunciating them. When combined with "a," "e," or "o," these two closed vowels, "i" and "u," form diphthongs, or gliding vowels, whose quick, single sounds more closely approximate the stronger open vowel sounds. The English phoneme "i" is most closely approximated in Spanish words like *hay* ("there is"). [The letter "h" is silent in Spanish.]

# Grammar Review

This quick presentation of basic grammar review is designed to refresh your memory about word types and uses. You probably haven't had the opportunity to do this since fourth grade, so enjoy!

This overview is by nature incomplete. It is intended to get you started, not convert you into a linguist. For further discussion, please consult one or more of the excellent text references listed at the end of this chapter. Also, consider taking an introductory conversational course in Spanish as soon as possible after reading this book.

# Word Typology

## Nouns

Nouns identify persons, places, or things. In Spanish, unlike in English, nouns (*sustantivos*) are almost always found in two forms—feminine and masculine. Feminine nouns normally (but not always) end in "a." Masculine nouns normally (but not always) end in "o." For example, *perra* means female dog; *perro* means male dog.

There are some exceptions to this general rule. Some nouns referring to people use the same form for females and males. *Artista* (artist), *modelo* (model), and *poeta* (poet) are examples of this phenomenon.

A few animal names like *jirafa* (giraffe) and *sapo* (toad) exist only in one gender. In these cases, Spanish speakers use the words *hembra* (female) and *macho* (male) to distinguish genders.

Generally, nouns ending in vowels are pluralized by just adding an "s," similar to how it generally happens in English. *Brazo/brazos* (arm/arms) is an example of this process. Nouns ending in consonants (except "z") are pluralized by adding "es." *Papel* and *papeles* (paper, singular and plural) are examples of this process. Nouns ending in "z" are pluralized by changing the "z" to "c" and adding "es." *Lápiz/lápices* (pencil/pencils) and *vez/veces* (time/times [per day, week, month, or year]) are examples of "z" changes.

## Articles

Articles (*artículos*) limit or particularize nouns. They may be definite (*determinados*), or specific, meaning "the," or indefinite (*indeterminados*), or general, meaning "a" or "an."

One fortunate aspect of the English language is that we only have one way to say "the." This is not the case with other languages like German (with six) and Spanish (with five). The Spanish forms of "the" include: *la* (feminine) and *el* (masculine), singular; and *las* (feminine) and *los* (masculine) plural; and *lo*. *Lo,* combined with a masculine singular adjective, expresses an abstract concept, as in *Es lo mismo para mí* (It's all the same to me). We'll leave *lo* alone for the rest of our discussion.

Examples of uses of definite articles include: *el* and *la paciente* (the patient, male and female), and *los* and *las terapeutas* (the therapists, male and female).

For linguistic reasons, it is difficult for Spanish speakers to enunciate two "a" phonemes together. As a result, words like *agua* (water) and *águila* (eagle) are feminine, but carry the definite article *el* instead of *la* in their singular forms. Hence, it is *el agua* in the singular form, but *las aguas* in the plural.

Be sure to use definite articles with nouns in conversation, when appropriate, just like with English. Remember, *la* usually precedes nouns ending in "a"; *el* precedes nouns ending in "o." Prominent exceptions include words like *la mano* (the hand) and *el síntoma* (the symptom), among others.

Indefinite articles are general in nature. In English, the indefinite articles are "a" and "an." In Spanish, they are: *un* (masculine) and *una* (feminine), singular; and *unos* (masculine) and *unas* (feminine), plural. Spanish indefinite articles agree in gender and number with the nouns and pronouns that they modify. Example: *Juan es un empleado.* (John is an employee.)

## Pronouns

Pronouns (*pronombres*) designate particular persons who are speaking or who are spoken to or about. While there are also prepositional, object, reflexive, and relative pronouns, this introduction addresses only the personal pronouns you are likely to need to know right away to communicate with Spanish-speaking patients.

The following outline delineates the personal pronouns in English and Spanish.

|  | **Singular** | **Plural** |
|---|---|---|
| 1st person: | I/*yo* | We/*nosotros* |
| 2nd person: | You/*usted* | You/*ustedes* |
| 3rd person: | He, she, it/*él/ella/ello* | They/*ellas/ellos* |

*Exercise #5: Read, practice, and memorize the following commonly used singular and plural personal pronouns in Spanish: first person* (yo, nosotros), *second person* (usted, ustedes), *and third person* (él, ella, ello, ellos, ellas). *We have ignored the second person familiar forms of "you,"* tu, vos, *and* vosotros *(used with children and persons with whom you are close or intimate), in favor of maintaining simplicity.*

## Adjectives

Adjectives (*adjetivos*) describe nouns and pronouns. Adjectives can address age, color, number, quality, quantity, weight, or other attributes that make nouns or pronouns more specific.

Adjectives most often come after nouns or pronouns in Spanish—the opposite of English. For example, "the big boy" in Spanish is *el niño grande*. One exception to this word order is possessive adjectives, like "my book," *mi libro*.

Possessive adjectives are important to learn in Spanish in order to communicate with patients. Possessive adjectives precede and agree with the nouns they modify in number. They include:

|  |  | Example |  |  |
|---|---|---|---|---|
| Mine: | *mi* or *mis* | (*ejemplo*): | My books: | *mis libros* |
| Your: | *su* or *sus* | *Ejemplo*: | Your arm: | *su brazo* |
| His, hers: | same as your | *Ejemplo*: | Her foot: | *su pie* |
| Our: | *nuestro/a* | *Ejemplo*: | Our house: | *nuestra casa* |

*Exercise #6: Read, practice, and memorize the Spanish possessive adjectives above. If you cannot memorize them, then tab your book for quick reference to them.*

## Verbs and Adverbs

A verb (*verbo*) is a word or words of action or of a state of being, forming the predicate that complements the subject in a sentence. Verb tenses are categorized according to their time frame—present, past, and future.

Spanish has fourteen verb tenses, English has six. Because it is utilized most of the time in conversation, we will deal exclusively with the present indicative tense at this level. The present indicative tense addresses the here and now. By using the present indicative tense, you can communicate effectively with your Spanish-speaking patients at the elemental level.

## Present Indicative Tense for Five Basic Verbs:

### Estar (to be)

| I | You (sing.) | He/she/it | We | You (plural) | They |
|---|---|---|---|---|---|
| *Estoy* | *Está* | *Está* | *Estamos* | *Están* | *Están* |

### Hacer (to do or make)

| I | You (sing.) | He/she/it | We | You (plural) | They |
|---|---|---|---|---|---|
| *Hago* | *Hace* | *Hace* | *Hacemos* | *Hacen* | *Hacen* |

### Ir (to go)

| I | You (sing.) | He/she/it | We | You (plural) | They |
|---|---|---|---|---|---|
| *Voy* | *Va* | *Va* | *Vamos* | *Van* | *Van* |

### Ser (to be)

| I | You (sing.) | He/she/it | We | You (plural) | They |
|---|---|---|---|---|---|
| *Soy* | *Ere* | *Es* | *Somos* | *Son* | *Son* |

### Tener (to have)

| I | You (sing.) | He/she/it | We | You (plural) | They |
|---|---|---|---|---|---|
| *Tengo* | *Tiene* | *Tiene* | *Tenemos* | *Tienen* | *Tienen* |

It is interesting to note that there are two infinitive verb forms of "to be" in Spanish—*estar* and *ser*. *Estar* is used to connote a physical or mental condition, or general health. It is the verb you will use when questioning your Spanish-speaking patients about illnesses. Example: Are you ill? *Está enferma?* [Note the hard accent on the final vowel "a."]

*Estar* is also used for geographic locations. San Diego is in California. *San Diego está en California.* It is used for emotions. I am sad. *Estoy triste. Estar* is also used for marital status. She's married to a European. *Está casada con un europeo.*

*Ser* is used to define or classify a person or thing. Examples: I am an American. *Soy estadounidense.* I am a doctor. *Soy médico. Ser* is used for events. The conference is here. *La conferencia es aquí.* Ser is also used to denote date and time. It's three o'clock. *Son las tres.* What time is it? *¿Qué hora es?*

If you cannot distinguish between *estar* and *ser* right away in Spanish conversation, use either one (at first). Spanish speakers will understand you. Then go back and review the rules on when to use the correct "to be" verb.

An adverb (*adverbio*) modifies a verb, adjective, or another adverb. In English, we often add "-ly" to a word to create an adverb. In Spanish, the suffix added is "-mente." For example: I am going quickly. *Voy rápidamente.*

---

*Exercise #7: Review, practice, and memorize the five basic Spanish verbs and their forms above. If you cannot memorize them, then tab your book for quick reference to them.*

---

## Prepositions and Prepositional Phrases

The main prepositions (*preposiciones*) in Spanish are: *a* (to), *de* (of), *para* (for), and *por* (by, for). Along with their objects (nouns, pronouns, or verbs), they form prepositional phrases.

Technically, *para* is used for the following reasons: comparison, destination, direction, employment, purpose, and when there is a targeted recipient. *Por* is used for agency, cause, choice, exchange, general location, motive, rate, reason, route, substitution, and time frame. *Por* tends to be retrofocused; *para* is forward-looking.

The following sentences illustrate some of the differences between *para* and *por*. Because the analog for both words is "for" in English, it is easy at first to mix them up, or to tend to overutilize *por*, since it is closest to "for." Don't worry too much about it. Spanish speakers will understand you even if you use the incorrect preposition.

> The book is for you. *El libro es para usted.* [targeted recipient]
> She works for UPS. *Ella trabaja para UPS.* [employment]
> The doctor's office is around here. *La oficina del médico está por aquí.* [general location]
> You go through San Antonio. *Usted pasa por San Antonio.* [route]

## Conjunctions

A conjunction (*conjunción*) is a word that links words, phrases, and clauses. Key coordinating conjunctions (connecting similar words) include "and" (*y*) and "but" (*pero*). An important subordinating conjunction (in this case showing cause and effect) is because (*porque*). [Note that the words "because" (*porque*) and "why" (*por qué*) are nearly identical in Spanish.]

## Pronunciation and Accents

There are a few pronunciation quirks in Spanish that you should be aware of. (Several of them have already been previewed in this book.) In Castilian Spanish, "z" is pronounced like "th." Throughout the rest of the Hispanic world, however, "z" is pronounced like an "s." I recommend that you pronounce "z" as "s." The letter "h" is silent in Spanish.

Several other Spanish pronunciation particulars bear mentioning. The letters "b" and "v" in Spanish are both pronounced like the English "b." The letter "j" in Spanish is pronounced like an "h." The "ll" in Spanish is pronounced like a "y." The letter "r" at the beginning of a word, and the double "rr" in the middle of a word, are trilled, like the sound of a motor revving, with your tongue vibrating rapidly behind your upper teeth at the front of the roof of your mouth.

Phonologically, Spanish speakers have difficulty beginning words with the letter "s." That is why Spanish speakers often pronounce "Spain" as "Espain."

Accents are used to show word syllable stress. Accents in Spanish are of two types—unwritten and written. Written accents always appear over vowels. In English, accents are unwritten, except for poetic metrical forms, such as iambic pentameter (five pairs of unstressed-stressed syllabi).

The rules for syllable stress in Spanish when there are no written accents are as follows. If a word ends in a consonant other than "n" or "s," the stress is over the last syllable. Example: *anda<u>dor</u>* (walker). If a word ends in a vowel, or "n" or "s," the stress is over the next-to-last (penultimate) syllable. Example: *pie<u>r</u>na* (leg).

For some time, a movement has been shaping to eliminate written accents in Spanish. In practice, they are seldom used by many, if not most, Hispanics in everyday writing.

# Basic Communicative Words and Phrases

## Titles:

1. Doctor, doctora: Dr.
2. Profesor, profesora: teacher
3. Señor/señora/señorita: Mr., Mrs., Ms.

## Greetings, Introductions, Farewells, and Other Basic Key Words:

1. *Buenos días.* Good morning.
2. *Buenas tardes.* Good afternoon.
3. *Buenas noches.* Good evening/good night.
4. *Hola.* Hi.
5. *Bienvenido.* Welcome.
6. *¿Cómo se llama usted?* What's your name?
7. *La dirección, el domicilio*: address
8. *Pase.* Come in.
9. *Pase al cuarto numero* _____, *por favor.* Please go to Room ___.
10. *Tome asiento, por favor.* Have a seat, please.
11. *¿Cómo está?* How are you?
12. *Bien.* Fine.
13. *No muy bien.* Not very well.

14. *Me duele el/la* _____. My _____ hurts.
15. *Por favor.* Please.
16. *Gracias.* Thanks.
17. *De nada.* You're welcome.
18. *Lo siento.* I'm sorry.
19. *Adiós.* Goodbye.
20. *Hasta mañana/la próxima visita.* Until tomorrow/the next appointment.

It is interesting to note that in Spanish, greetings like "good morning," "good afternoon," and "good night" are said in plural forms. For example, *buenos días* literally translates into "good mornings." In other Latin languages like Portuguese, *bom dia* is literally analogous to "good morning" in English, as are *boa tarde* and *boa noite* (good afternoon and good night).

### Numbers:

*Uno:* one
*Dos:* two
*Tres:* three
*Cuatro:* four
*Cinco:* five
*Seis:* six
*Siete:* seven
*Ocho:* eight
*Nueve:* nine
*Diez:* ten
*Once:* eleven
*Doce:* twelve
*Trece:* thirteen
*Catorce:* fourteen
*Quince:* fifteen
*Dieciseis:* sixteen ["10 + 6"]
*Diecisiete:* seventeen
*Dieciocho:* eighteen

*Diecinueve:* nineteen
*Veinte:* twenty
*Trienta:* thirty
*Cuarenta:* forty
*Cincuenta:* fifty
*Sesenta:* sixty
*Setenta:* seventy
*Ochenta:* eighty
*Noventa:* ninety
*Cien:* one hundred
*Mil:* one thousand
*Millón:* one million

## Day and time landmarks:

*Lunes:* Monday
*Martes:* Tuesday
*Miércoles:* Wednesday
*Jueves:* Thursday
*Viernes:* Friday
*Sábado:* Saturday
*Domingo:* Sunday

*Enero:* January
*Febrero:* February
*Marzo:* March
*Abril:* April
*Mayo:* May
*Junio:* June
*Julio:* July
*Agosto:* August
*Septiembre:* September
*Octubre:* October
*Noviembre:* November
*Diciembre:* December

*Hoy:* today
*Mañana:* tomorrow
*Ayer:* yesterday
*La semana pasada:* last week
*La semana que viene:* next week

*La mañana:* morning
*La tarde:* afternoon
*La noche:* night

*La hora:* hour
*El minuto:* minute
*El segundo:* second [unit of time and ordinal number]

## Colors:

*Amarillo:* yellow
*Azul:* blue
*Blanco:* white
*Gris:* gray
*Marrón:* brown
*Negro:* black
*Rojo:* red
*Rosado:* pink
*Verde:* green

## Hair colors and traits:

*Morena/o:* dark-haired
*Pelirroja/o:* red-head
*Rubia/o:* blonde
*Cabello:* hair on one's head
*Pelo púbico:* pubic hair
*Vello:* body hair

## Dimensions and attributes:

*Alta/o:* high, tall
*Altura:* height

*Ancha/o:* wide
*Áspera/o:* rough
*Baja/o:* low, short (height)
*Clara/o:* light
*Corta/o:* short (length)
*Delgada/o:* thin build
*Derecha/o:* right
*Dura/o:* hard
*Elevada/o:* raised
*Gorda/o:* heavy build
*Grande:* large
*Grasa/o:* oily (skin)
*Izquierda/o:* left
*Larga/o:* long (height)
*Mojada/o:* wet
*Oscura/o:* dark
*Pequeña/o:* small
*Pesa/o:* weight
*Plana/o:* flat
*Seca/o:* dry
*Suave:* smooth
*Volúmen:* volume

### Transportation:

*A pie:* on foot
*En autobús:* by bus
*En bicicleta:* by bike
*En coche:* by car
*En taxi:* by taxi

---

*Exercise #8: Using what you have learned so far, translate the following dialogue between a patient and a nurse practitioner into Spanish. Use Spanglish and/or English to make sentences complete, as needed. Good luck!*

---

Patient: Good morning, Ms. Smith.
 Nurse: Hi, Mrs. Álvarez. Come in. How are you today?
Patient: My right leg hurts.
 Nurse: I'm sorry to hear that. Come in. Please go to Room 7.
Patient: Thanks.
 Nurse: You're welcome.

## SUMMARY

Spanish and English differ substantially in terms of linguistics and phonetics. Spanish is Latin-based; English is Germanic. In terms of grammar,
there are 14 verb tenses in Spanish, compared to six in English. Spanish
vowel sounds are straightforward compared to English—what you see
is literally what you get. Mastering key words, phrases, and basic verbs
in the present indicative tense helps foster smoother communications
between health care providers and Spanish-speaking patients and their
significant others. Translator intervention is still required for critical care-
related conversations like obtaining informed consent, communicating a
patient's diagnosis, and perioperative communications.

## DISCUSSION QUESTIONS AND ACTIVITIES

1. Does the pervasive use of Spanish words and phrases in the
   media in the United States make it easier to learn elemental
   Spanish?
2. There are five basic vowel sounds in Spanish. How many vowel
   sounds are there in English?
3. What strategies and tactics help you learn and master new words
   and phrases? After one week, how many Spanish words and
   phrases from this and preceding chapters have you mastered?
4. As you interact with Spanish speakers, try to distinguish regional
   pronunciation and accents.
5. Use a comprehensive Spanish dictionary or verb table and
   conjugate the Spanish verb *hablar* (from the Chapter 1 vocabulary list) in the present indicative tense.

# REFERENCES AND READINGS

1. Kendris C. *501 Spanish verbs,* 4th ed. 1996, Hauppauge NY: Barron's Educational Series.
2. Lunn PV, DeCesaris JA. *Investigación de gramatica.* 1992, Boston, MA: Heinle & Heinle.
3. Reyes G. *Cómo escribir bien en español,* 3rd ed. 2001, Arco Libros: Madrid, Spain.
4. Spinelli E. *English grammar for students of Spanish,* 3rd ed. 1994, Olivia and Hill Press: Ann Arbor, MI.
5. Teschner RV. *Camino oral,* 2nd ed. 2000, New York: McGraw-Hill.

# Chapter 5

# The Medical Nitty-Gritty– You Can Do This!

*Clinical health care delivery has five basic components: (1) examination (including history-taking, physical examination, and physical and mental tests and measurements); (2) evaluation (analysis of examination findings); (3) diagnosis; (4) prognosis; and (5) either appropriate intervention, or referring the patient for further study, care, and/or patient education. This chapter explores key words and phrases needed by health care professionals to carry out these processes with Spanish-speaking patients. Words that have appeared elsewhere in the text are not repeated in other sections, but are indexed alphabetically in English and Spanish in Appendix A.*

## OBJECTIVES

1. Familiarize yourself with key Spanish words and phrases used in clinical health care delivery.
2. Recognize the close similarities between many Latin-based and co-opted Spanish and English language medical words and phrases.
3. Incorporate English and/or Spanglish as needed into health care-related conversations with Spanish-speaking patients in order to communicate better with them.
4. Practice everyday conversations between English-speaking health care providers and Spanish-speaking patients and significant others.

5. Consider taking a formal Spanish language course at a college or university to build on what you have learned thus far.

## VOCABULARY

*La/el ayudante* (aide)

*Beber* (to drink)

*El bolígrafo* (pen)

*Comer* (to eat)

*La/el compañera/o* (companion)

*Cuando* (when)

*Cuánto* (how many/much)

*Doler* (to ache or hurt)

*El dolor* (pain)

*Donde* (where)

*La esposa, el esposo* (spouse)

*Ésta/éste/esto*

*Examinar* (to examine)

*La hija, el hijo* (daughter, son)

*El ingreso* (admission)

*Las instrucciones al paciente* (patient instructions)

*Lo más pronto posible* (as soon as possible)

*La mañana* (morning)

*La medicación, el medicamento* (medication)

*La medicina* (medicine)

*La medicina gerenciada* (managed care)

*Mover* (to move)

*Necesitar* (to need)

*La nieta, el nieto* (grandchild)

*La noche* (night)

*Paciente ambulatorio* (outpatient)

*Paciente hospitalizado* (in-patient)

*La/el recepcionista* (receptionist)

*Rellenar* (to fill out [papers])

*La tarde* (afternoon, late)

*Temprano* (early)

*Tomar* (to take)

*Trabajar* (to work)

This chapter addresses basic communication between primary clinical health care providers and their patients. This chapter and the next take a different approach than the previous three chapters in that they mainly contain easy-to-use, alphabetized reference lists of key clinical terms in Spanish.

Clinical health care delivery has five key components (or processes). The first is patient intake, including an initial greeting (some of the words and phrases for which we have already covered in the preceding chapter), filling out necessary paperwork, taking a relevant patient history, and the physical examination. The history-taking and physical process include the important steps of ascertaining the patient's chief complaint (or complaints) and ordering or recommending pertinent tests and measurements, such as diagnostic imaging and laboratory studies.

The second major clinical health care delivery process is the evaluation of examination and test findings. This is when the primary health care clinician synthesizes subjective and objective data into potential diagnoses. This phase of clinical health care delivery is somewhat analogous, at least in structure, to ascertaining the reasonable potential interventions in order to share them with a patient during the informed consent disclosure process.

The third process is to reach a precise and accurate diagnosis. Experienced expert clinicians can do this more quickly than novice clinicians because they categorize data into schema and subconsciously discard unnecessary information along the way.

The fourth process is to develop a prognosis for each patient under care. The final step is intervention—treatment, referral to another health care professional, instructions about home and self care (*instrucciones al paciente*), and patient education (*educación médica para el paciente*). Managed care (*medicina gerenciada*) care has profoundly affected the amount of time that providers have to work with patients. Providers should be cognizant of studies that conclude that non-English-speaking patients are less satisfied with health care delivery than their English-speaking counterparts.

Try to familiarize yourself with the sampling of basic communicative words below. Remember to precede nouns with their definite articles *la* or *el* in conversation when appropriate.

### Patient Intake

*La/el ayudante:* aide

*El bolígrafo:* pen

*La/el compañera/o:* companion

*Dar de alta:* discharge from hospital

*La dirección, el domicilio:* address

*Doler* (to hurt)

*El dolor* (pain)

*La fiebre* (fever)

*¿Habla inglés/español?* Do you speak English/Spanish?

*El mareo* (dizziness)

*¿Necesita un bolígrafo/una lápiz?* Do you need a pen/pencil?

*Por favor, rellene este papel.* Please fill out this paper.

*La/el recepcionista:* receptionist

*Los síntomas* (symptoms)

*Usted ha llegado tarde/temprano.* You've arrived late/early.

*Le veremos lo más pronto possible.* We'll see you as soon as possible.

*Los vómitos* (vomiting)

## What Is the Patient's Problem?

*¿Cuál problema médico tiene?* What is your medical problem?

*¿Tiene dolor?* Are you in pain?

*¿Dónde le duele?* Where does it hurt?

*¿Cuánto tiempo?* How long?

*¿Algunos otros síntomas?* Any other symptoms?

*¿Cuáles son?* What are they?

*¿Puede beber/comer?* Are you able to drink/eat?

*¿Tiene mareo?* Are you dizzy?

*¿Tiene fiebre?* Do you have a fever?

*¿Ha vomitado?* Have you vomited?

## Medical and Social History-Taking

*¿Qué causó sus síntomas?* What caused your symptoms?

*¿Ha tenido estos síntomas antes?* Have you had these symptoms before?

*¿Cuándo?* When?

*Apunte con un dedo dónde le duele.* Point with one finger where it hurts.

*¿Dónde trabaja?* Where do you work?

*¿Cuántas personas en su familia nuclear?* How many persons in your nuclear family?

*La/el esposa/o:* spouse

*La/el hija/o:* daughter/son

*La/el nieta/o:* grandchild

## Systems Review and Physical Examination

*Quítese por favor su...* Please remove your...

*El abrigo:* coat

*La blusa:* blouse

*Los calcetines:* socks

*La camisa:* shirt

*La falda:* skirt

*Los pantalones:* pants

*El sujetador:* bra

*El vestido:* dress

*Los zapatos:* shoes

*Póngase esta bata, por favor.* Please put on this robe.


*Me gustaría examinarle.* I would like to examine you.

*Mueve su _____, por favor.* Move your _____ please.

*Así:* like this

*Abajo:* down

*Adelante:* forward

*Adentro:* inside

*Afuera:* outside

*A la derecha:* to the right

*A la izquierda:* to the left

*Arriba:* up

*Hacia atrás:* backward

*¿Cómo se dice...?* How do you say...?

*Perdóneme:* Pardon me

*Sentir dormido:* To feel numb

*Tener cosquillas/hormigueo:* To feel a tingling sensation

*Ya está.* That's enough.


*La cabeza:* head

*La cara:* face

*El ojo:* eye

*La oreja:* ear

*El tímpano:* eardrum

*La nariz:* nose

*La boca:* mouth

*Los labios:* lips

*El/los diente(s):* tooth, teeth
*Las encías:* gums
*La lengua:* tongue
*El cuello:* neck
*El hombro:* shoulder
*El brazo:* arm
*El codo:* elbow
*El antebrazo:* forearm
*La muñeca:* wrist
*La mano:* hand
*Los dedo(s):* fingers
*El/los pulgar(es):* thumb(s)
*El pecho:* chest
*La costilla:* rib
*La cintura:* waist
*El ombligo:* navel
*La cadera:* hip
*Las nalgas:* buttocks
*El muslo:* thigh
*La rodilla:* knee
*La espinilla:* shin
*La pantorrilla:* calf
*El tobillo:* ankle
*El pie:* foot
*El/los dedo(s) del pie:* toe(s)
*El dedo gordo:* great toe

*El cráneo:* skull
*La mandíbula:* jaw
*La clavícula:* collarbone
*El humero:* humerus
*El radio:* radius
*El cúbito:* ulna
*Los carpos:* wrist bones

*Las falanges:* phalanges (hands and feet)

*El esternón:* sternum

*El omóplato:* scapula [also escápula]

*La columna vertebral:* vertebral column

*El hueso ilíaco:* ilium

*El fémur:* femur

*La rótula:* patella


*El cerebro:* brain

*La garganta:* throat

*El corazón:* heart

*Las arterias:* arteries

*Las venas:* veins

*Los pulmones:* lungs

*El hígado:* liver

*La vesícula biliar:* gallbladder

*El estómago:* stomach

*El páncreas:* pancreas

*El bazo:* spleen

*El intestino delgado:* small intestine

*El intestino grueso:* large intestine

*El ano:* anus

*Los riñones:* kidneys

*La vejiga:* urinary bladder

### Diagnoses and Interventions

*La ampolla:* blister

*El análisis de laboratorio:* lab test

*La apendicítis:* appendicitis

*El cáncer:* cancer

*El cardenal:* bruise [also *la contusión*]

*La consulta:* consultation

*La coordinación:* coordination

*La fractura:* fracture

*Haga estos ejercicios.* Do these exercises. *Muéstreme que los sabe hacer.* Show me that you know how to do them.

*La hepatitis:* hepatitis

*La infección:* infection

*La inyección:* injection

*La laceración:* laceration

*La medicación, el medicamento:* medication

*La medicina:* medicine

*La radiografía:* x-ray

*La receta:* prescription

*La recomendación:* referral

*La repetición de una receta:* prescription refill

*La sala de rayos X:* x-ray department

*Tome esta medicina dos veces al día.* Take this medicine twice a day.

*Use esta crema/pomada.* Use this cream/ointment.

## Specialty Care

### AIDS:

*Los antiretrovirales:* antiretroviral drugs

*El SIDA (sindrome inmunodeficiencia adquirida):* AIDS

*El VIH (virus de inmunodeficiencia humano):* HIV

### Geriatrics:

*¿Cuántos años tiene usted?* How old are you?

*¿Vive sola/o?* Do you live alone?

*¿Tiene amigas/os o familia cerca?* Do you have friends or family nearby?

*¿Conduce un coche/carro?* Do you drive?

*¿Fuma cigarillos?¿Cuántos al día?* Do you smoke cigarettes? How many per day?

*¿Bebe alcohol?* Do you drink alcohol?

*¿Algunos problemas con dormir?* Any problems sleeping?

*¿Tiene problemas cuidarse/levantarse y abajarse?* Do you have any problem taking care of yourself/getting up or down?

*¿Se ha caído recientemente?* Have you fallen recently?

*¿Tiene problemas con orinar o evacuar?* Do you have any problems with urination or defecation?

*¿Cuántos medicamentos toma cada día?* How many medications do you take daily?

*Tiene o ha tenido _____?* Do you have or have you had _____?

*Artritis:* arthritis

*Colesterol elevado:* high cholesterol

*Diabetes:* diabetes

*Enfermedad de riñones:* kidney disease

*Glaucoma:* glaucoma

*Infarto de miocardio:* myocardial infarction

*Tensión alta:* high blood pressure

*Tuberculosis:* tuberculosis

### Men's Health:

*El condón:* condom

*La eyaculación:* ejaculation

*La erección:* erection

*La masturbación:* masturbation

*El pene:* penis

*La próstata:* prostate

*El semen:* semen

*Los testículos:* testicles

*La uretra:* urethra

*La vasectomía:* vasectomy

### Pediatrics:

*La/el adolescente:* adolescent

*La anorexia:* anorexia

*El asma:* asthma

*La/el bebé:* baby

*El desorden de deficiencia de atención debido a la hiperactividad:* attention deficit hyperactivity disorder

*La dislexia:* dyslexia

*La escoliosis:* scoliosis

*La niña pequeña/el niño pequeño:* toddler

*Las paperas:* mumps

*El sarampión:* measles

*La vacunación:* immunization

*La varicela:* chicken pox

## Pregnancy:

*El aborto involuntario:* miscarriage

*El aborto voluntario:* abortion

*La cesárea:* Caesarean section

*Dar luz:* give birth

*Dar pecho:* breastfeed

*El dolor de espalda:* low back pain

*Los dolores del parto:* labor pains

*Embarazada/encinta:* pregnant

*El embarazo:* pregnancy [not *preñez*, which means "animal pregnancy," but is sometimes used inappropriately for human pregnancy]

*La nausea:* nausea

*El período/la regla:* period

*El peso:* weight

*¿Se le ha roto la fuente?* Has your water broken?

## Psychology:

*La depresión*: depression

*La/el deprimida/o*: depressed

*La esquizofrenia*: schizoprenia

*Maníaca/o*: manic

*La neurosis*: neurosis

*Nerviosa/o*: nervous

*Los problemas emocionales:* emotional problems

*Los problemas psiquiátricos:* psychiatric problems

*La psicosis:* psychosis

*El trastorno bipolar:* bipolar disorder

*El trastorno obsesivocompulsivo:* obsessive-compulsive disorder

**Women's Health:**

*La cérvix:* cervix

*El ciclo menstrual:* menstrual cycle

*El clítoris:* clitoris

*El control de la natalidad:* birth control

*El mamograma:* mammogram

*La mastectomía:* mastectomy

*La menopausia:* menopause

*La menstruación:* menstruation

*El orgasmo:* orgasm

*El examen Papanicolau (el Pap):* Pap smear

*El pezón:* nipple

*La secreción vaginal:* vaginal discharge

*El seno:* breast

*Los tubos de falopio:* Fallopian tubes

*El úterò:* uterus

*La vagina:* vagina

---

*Exercise #9: Using this book and a Spanish dictionary as needed, translate the following dialogue into Spanish.*

---

Receptionist: Hi! Good morning. Are you Mrs. Barba?

Sra. Barba: Yes, I am. I have an appointment with Dr. Scott at 10 o'clock.

Receptionist: OK. Have a seat, please.

[Three minutes later]

Receptionist: Please fill out this paper.

Sra. Barba: OK. Do you have a pen? Thanks!

Dr. Scott: Mrs. Barba? Welcome! Please go into Room 8.

[Three minutes later]

Dr. Scott: What medical problem do you have?

Sra. Barba: Low back pain.

Dr. Scott: What are your symptoms?

Sra. Barba: Pain in my left leg, and numbness and tingling in my left foot.

> Dr. Scott:    I would like to examine you. Please take off your blouse, bra, skirt, and shoes, and put on this gown. I'll be back in a minute.

## SUMMARY

The processes of patient care include patient intake, history and physical examination, diagnosis, prognosis, and intervention. To interact effectively with Spanish-speaking patients and families, it is important to familiarize yourself with an array of basic patient care-related words, phrases, and questions. This chapter has introduced some 236 of them. Because so many medical words worldwide are Latin-based, more medical words are identical or similar in English and Spanish. Familiarizing yourself with them and practicing them will help facilitate self-confidence and better communications between you and Spanish speakers. Remember to "apply the mortar" (fill in gaps in Spanish with English words and phrases) when you don't know how to say words and phrases in Spanish.

## DISCUSSION QUESTIONS

1. Which words and phrases presented in this chapter are identical in Spanish and English? What is probably still different about the presentation of these words to Spanish-speaking patients by English-speaking health care professionals?

2. The chapter presents an array of practice-specific medical words and phrases in Spanish. Ascertain which additional key words and phrases are pertinent to your particular practice and create a list (with Spanish translations from a dictionary or the Internet) in the inside back cover of the book for ready reference.

3. Were you surprised in Exercise #9 that it was relatively easy to translate a passage between providers and patient from English into Spanish? Is this direction of translation easier, harder, or no different for the Spanish words that you have already mastered?

4. So many American English medical words, especially those involving pharmaceuticals, have been co-opted into other languages. Why do you think this is so?

5. There is evidence from the Weech-Maldonado study listed in the references below that non-English-speaking patients are

relatively dissatisfied with health care in the United States. What steps can and do you take in your practice to make them more satisfied with care? Do you think that dissatisfied patients are more likely to sue providers for health care malpractice?

## REFERENCES AND READINGS

1. Acosta-Sariego JR. Atención integral de la salud como cuestión ética. www.panorama.sld.cu [discussion of managed care].
2. Weech-Maldonado R, Elliott M, Morales L, Spritzer K, Marshall G, Hays R. Health plan effects on patient assessments of Medicaid managed care among racial/ethnic minorities. Journal of General Internal Medicine. 2004; 19(2): 136–145. [Non-English speakers report worse experiences with health care service delivery than English speaking patients.]
3. Spanish Today. *San Antonio Express News.* Jan. 28, 2007, 9J. [Differentiates between selected Spanish and English words that look alike but have different meanings—*rebatir* (to refute) and *reembolsar* (to give or receive a rebate); great ongoing series.]
4. Google.es. [Google.es is Spain's version of Google. It is an excellent, up-to-the-minute resource for translating difficult words and phrases into Spanish. To find a word in Spanish, just type the word in English and add the word "Spanish" after it.]

# Chapter 6

# Focus on Rehabilitation

*Physical rehabilitation entails the restoration and improvement of patient functional abilities after injury or illness. Professionals directly involved in physical rehabilitation include, among others, physical medicine physician specialists; rehabilitation nurses; occupational, physical, and speech therapists; orthotists and prosthetists; social workers and vocational rehabilitation specialists; and assistants and support professionals. A substantial proportion of the population in the United States is Spanish speaking. This means that rehabilitation professionals must be competent in elemental Spanish in order to converse with these patients in their primary language, optimizing their recovery potential.*

## OBJECTIVES

1. Learn and use basic rehabilitation terms in Spanish with Spanish-speaking patients.
2. Develop and use pain questions in Spanish for appropriate patients.
3. Communicate critical patient safety instructions to Spanish-speaking rehabilitation patients regarding crutch walking and fall prevention.
4. Carry out patient home-exercise education using relevant words and phrases in Spanish.
5. Develop and refine a crutch-walking instruction sheet for Spanish-speaking patients.

## VOCABULARY

*Las actividades de la vida cotidiana* (activities of daily living)

*¿Cuánto tiempo?* How long?

*De frente* (front view)

*Detrás* (back view)

*El dibujo* (drawing)

*Enséñeme:* Show me.

*La escala del dolor* (pain scale)

*La fase* (phase)

*La intensidad* (intensity)

*Más* (more)

*Menos* (less)

*La movilidad* (mobility)

*Los palos* (sticks)

*Las preguntas* (questions)

*El peso sobre la pierna débil* (weight-bearing)

*La silla de ruedas* (wheelchair)

Each year, millions of patients are affected by potentially debilitating medical conditions caused by disease and injury, such as amputations, cancer, fractures, heart attacks, paralysis, and strokes, among a myriad of others. In fact, since January 2005, Brooke Army Medical Center, in San Antonio, Texas, has operated the world's largest amputee care center, treating the tens of thousands of American military service-members who have suffered traumatic amputations in the Iraq and Afghanistan wars. The Amputee Care Center (ACC) has a three-phase mission: to provide interdisciplinary team continuity of care from patient intake through surgery to inpatient and outpatient rehabilitation. The stated goal for every patient is functional independence outside of the hospital environment. The ACC contains the world's largest physical and occupational therapy department—financed entirely through private donations. For more information, and a photo array of the ACC, please visit its website at www.bamc.amedd.army.mil/ACC.

---

*Exercise #10: Find all of the medical terms in the introductory paragraph above about debilitating medical conditions and Brooke Army Medical Center's new Amputee Care Center. How many of these terms are you already familiar with in Spanish? Write them down in a journal as you go along. I count at least thirty-two words. Impressive!*

---

Physical rehabilitation entails the restoration and improvement of patient functional abilities after injury or illness. Professionals directly involved in physical rehabilitation include, among others, physical medicine physician specialists; rehabilitation nurses; occupational, physical, and speech therapists; orthotists and prosthetists; social workers and vocational rehabilitation specialists; and assistants and support professionals. A substantial proportion of the population in the United States is Spanish speaking. This means that rehabilitation professionals must be competent in elemental Spanish in order to converse with these patients in their primary language, optimizing their recovery potential.

This chapter presents an array of medical terms in selected areas of patient rehabilitation. It is intended to provide a starting point, from which you hopefully will be enticed into undertaking further formal study of the Spanish language. Many colleges and universities even offer focused night courses in medical Spanish.

## Pain Questions (Preguntas sobre el dolor)

*¿Tiene dolor ahora?* Are you in pain now?

*¿Cuánto tiempo hace que lo tiene?* How long have you had it?

*Es _____?* Is it _____?

> *Pesado:* dull
>
> *Agudo:* sharp
>
> *Leve:* mild
>
> *Moderado:* moderate
>
> *Severo:* severe
>
> *Local:* local
>
> *Extendido:* radiating
>
> *Constante:* constant
>
> *Me va y me viene:* intermittent
>
> *Quemante:* burning

*¿Qué intensidad tiene su dolor, desde uno (lo menos) hasta diez (lo más posible)?* How intense is your pain, on a scale of one (least) to ten (most)?

*¿Es peor el dolor cuando se sienta o cuando se levanta?* Is the pain worse when you sit or stand?

*¿Le despierta el dolor por la noche cuando está durmiendo?* Does your pain wake you up at night when you are sleeping?

*Descríbame su dolor, en sus propias palabras.* Describe your pain in your own words.

*El dibujo anatómico.* Pain drawing.

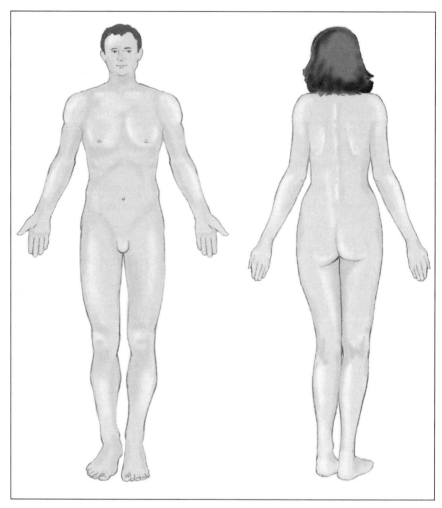

Figure 6.1   *De frente* (frontal view)                   *Detrás* (back view)

*¿Dónde le duele?* Where does it hurt?

*Marque el área con una "x".* Mark the area with an "x".

Pain Scale (La escala del dolor)

Put an "x" where your pain belongs. (Ponga una "x" donde le pertenece el dolor.)

| 0 | 1 | 2 | 3 | 4 | 5 | 6 | 7 | 8 | 9 | 10 |
|---|---|---|---|---|---|---|---|---|---|---|

| No pain | Mild | | | | Moderate | | | | | Severe |
|---|---|---|---|---|---|---|---|---|---|---|
| (Ninguno) | (Leve) | | | | (Moderado) | | | | | (Severo) |

## Special Tests and Measurements

### *La valoración muscular (or el exámen de los músculos):* muscle testing

Hint: Whether your patients speak English, Spanish, or any other language, consider manually demonstrating the desired movements for patients before they attempt them.

*Mueva el brazo, la pierna, etc., así, por favor. Gracias.* Move your arm, leg, etc., like this, please. Thanks.

*La flexión* (or *doblar*): flexion

*La extensión* (or *poner derecho*): extension

*La abducción:* abduction

*La aducción:* adduction

*La rotación:* rotation

  *Externa:* external

  *Interna:* internal

*Mantenga esta posición, por favor.* Please hold this position.

*Fuerza:* strength

  *Normal:* normal

  *Buena:* good

  *Regular:* fair

  *Débil:* weak

  *Vestigio:* trace

  *Cero:* zero

*Aprete contra mi mano con toda fuerza.* Push against my hand with all your strength. *Cuidado. No debe doler.* Careful. It shouldn't hurt.

### Muscle Strength Grades (Los grados musculares)[1]

| Grado | Fuerza |
|-------|--------|
| 1 | *Normal* |
| 2 | *Buena* |
| 3 | *Regular* |
| 4 | *Débil* |
| 5 | *Vestigios* |
| 0 | *Cero* |

## Gait, Functional, and Postural Analyses *(Análisis de la forma de andar, de la función y de la postura)*

*Andar:* to walk [also *caminar*]

*Atar los zapatos:* to tie one's shoes

*Balancear los brazos:* arm swing

*Bañarse:* to take a bath

*Cepillar los dientes:* brush teeth

*La cifosis:* kyphosis

*La cojera:* limp

*El equilibrio:* balance

*La fase de contacto:* stance phase

*Lentamente:* slowly

*Levantarse:* to get up

*Limpiar la casa:* to do housework

*La línea recta a plomo:* plumb line

*La lordosis:* lordosis

*Los pasos:* steps

  *Más grandes:* bigger

  *Más pequenos:* smaller

  *Las pisadas perfectas:* perfect steps

*La pelvis:* pelvis

*Rápidamente:* quickly

*Recto:* straight

*Sentarse:* to sit down

*La silla de ruedas* (wheelchair)

*El tronco:* trunk

### Therapeutic Exercises *(Ejercicios terapéuticos)*

*Aeróbico:* aerobic (exercise)

*El alargamiento:* lengthening

*El agonista:* agonist

*El antagonista:* antagonist

*Bajar:* to lower

*La bicicleta:* bicycle

*La cadena abierta:* open chain
*La cadena cerrada:* closed chain
*Cardiovascular:* cardiovascular
*La circulación:* circulation
*La contracción muscular:* muscle contraction
   *Isométrica:* isometric
   *Isotónica:* isotonic
*Los ejercicios para hacer en casa:* home exercises
*El estabilizador:* stabilizer (muscle)
*Estirar:* to stretch
*Exhalar:* exhale
*Las extremidades:* extremities
*La fatiga muscular:* muscle fatigue
*Fortalecer:* to strengthen
*La fuerza dinámica:* dynamic strength
*La fuerza estática:* static strength
*Inspirar:* inhale
*Junto:* together
*El levantamiento de pesas:* weightlifting
*Levantar:* to raise
*La longitud:* length
*El músculo esquelético:* skeletal muscle
*El músculo estriado:* striated muscle
*Las pesas:* weights
*Relajar:* to relax
*Las repeticiones:* repetitions
*La resistencia:* endurance, resistance
*La rueda de ardilla:* treadmill [literally "squirrel wheel"]
*Separado:* apart
*El sinergista:* synergist
*La velocidad:* speed
*El bíceps (braquial):* Biceps
*El cuádriceps:* Quadriceps
*El deltoides:* Deltoids

*El esternocleidomastoideo:* Sternocleidomastoidus

*El gastrocnemio:* Gastrocnemius

*El gluteo mayor:* Gluteus maximus

*Los intercostales:* Intercostals

*El pectoral mayor:* Pectoralis major

*El recto del abdomen:* Rectus abdominus

*El trapezio:* Trapezius

*El tríceps:* Triceps

*Enfoque en ejercicios para la espalda:* Focus on back exercises

1. *Hábitos deseables para la buena salud:* Good habits for good health
   a. *Baje de peso.* Lose weight.
   b. *Beba con moderación.* Drink in moderacion.
   c. *Haga ejercicios.* Exercise.
   d. *No fume.* Don't smoke.
2. *Ejercicios:* Exercises
   a. *El estiramiento:* stretching
   b. *La inclinación pelvica:* pelvic tilt
   c. *La extensión:* extension
   d. *La flexión:* flexion
3. *Consejo practico: buena mecánica del cuerpo para proteger la espalda* (Practical advice: good body mechanics to protect the back)
   a. *Duerma en un colchón firme de alta calidad.* Sleep on a high-quality, firm mattress.
   b. *Levántese y bájese sin torcer la espalda.* Get up and down without twisting your back.
   c. *Suba objetos pesados con cuidado.* Lift heavy objects with care.[2]
      i. *Pruebe un objeto para saber cuanto pesa antes de levantarlo.* Test an object's weight before lifting it.
      ii. *Con los pies un poco mas apartados que los hombros, flexiona solamente las caderas y rodillas (un poco), no la espalda.* With feet a little more than shoulder-width apart, bend just your hips and knees a little, but not your back.
      iii. *Mantenga el objeto cerca de su cuerpo.* Keep the object close to your body.

iv. *Mantenga la espalda en una curvatura natural mientras levanta un objeto.* Keep your back in a neutral position when lifting any object.

v. *No se tuerza la cintura.* Don't twist at the waist while lifting.

## Modalities and Manual Procedures *(Modalidades y procedemientos manuales)*

*El baño de remolino:* whirlpool bath

*La compresa caliente:* hot pack

*La compresa fría:* cold pack

*La estimulación eléctrica:* electrical stimulation

*El estímulo eléctrico transcutáneo del nervio:* transcutaneous electrical nerve stimulation

*El gel analgésico:* analgesic gel

*El hielo:* ice

*La manipulación:* manipulation

*El masaje:* massage

*La movilización:* mobilization

*La parafina:* paraffin

*La piscina terapéutica:* therapy pool

*La posición abierta:* open-pack (joint) position

*La posición cerrada:* close-pack (joint) position

*La tracción:* traction

　*Cervical:* cervical

　*Lumbar:* lumbar

*El ultrasonido:* ultrasound

*Andando con muletas:* crutch walking

*La caída:* fall

*Las muletas:* crutches

*Las muletas axilares:* axillary crutches

*Las muletas del antebrazo:* forearm crutches

*La neuropraxia axilar:* axillary nerve damage

*Enfoque en usar las muletas axilares.* Focus on using axillary crutches.

1. *Medidas:* measurements
   a. *Seis pulgadas al lado de los pies:* six inches out from the feet
   b. *Un poco al frente de cada pie:* a little in front of each foot
   c. *Dos pulgadas debajo del hueco axilar:* two inches below the armpit
   d. *Adjuste los sostenes para tener 15 hasta 25 grados de flexión en el codo.* Adjust the handgrips so that there are 15–25 degrees of flexion at the elbows.
2. *Levantándose:* getting up
   a. *Muletas juntas en el lado débil:* crutches together on the weak side
   b. *Aprete los dos sostenes con la mano del lado débil.* Grasp the handgrips with the weak-side hand.
   c. *Ponga la otra mano sobre la silla.* Put the other hand on the seat.
   d. *Empújese arriba con las dos manos.* Push up with both hands.
   e. *Enderezca la pierna fuerte.* Straighten out the strong lower limb.
3. *Sentándose:* sitting down
   a. *Muletas juntas en el lado débil:* crutches together on the weak side
   b. *Aprete los dos sostenes con la mano del lado débil.* Grasp the handgrips with the weak side hand
   c. *Ponga la otra mano sobre la silla.* Put the other hand on the seat.
   d. *Abajese usando las dos manos y la pierna fuerte.* Descend using your two hands and your strong leg.
   e. *Cuidado con la pierna debil.* Be careful with the injured leg.
4. *Esté seguro que la silla esté apoyada.* Make sure the chair is supported.
5. *Caminando:* walking
   a. *Apoye el peso con sus manos.* Support your weight with your hands.
   b. *Peso sobre la pierna débil* (weight bearing)
      i. *Ningún peso:* no weight
      ii. *Peso parcial:* partial weight
      iii. *Peso completo:* full weight

    c. *¡Cuidado con el equilibrio!* Be careful with your balance!

    d. *No aprete las almohadillas axilares contra los sobacos.* Don't put pressure on the armpits with the axillary pads.

    e. *Si va a caerse, tire las muletas afuera para que no se caiga encima de ellas.* If you start to fall, throw your crutches out to the sides, so you don't fall on them.

6. *Pisando en escaleras o bordos:* walking on steps or curbs.

    a. *Orden arriba: pierna fuerte, pierna débil, muletas.* Order up: strong first, then weak, then crutches.

    b. *Orden abajo: muletas, pierna débil, pierna fuerte.* Order down: crutches, strong leg, weak leg.

## SUMMARY

There are thousands of specialized rehabilitation-related words and phrases in English and Spanish. The complexity of such terms and their translation is made more facile in part because many of these words and phrases share common Latin origins, especially the names for muscles and nerves. Pictorial diagrams may aid communications, where English-speaking health care professionals and Spanish-speaking patients cannot otherwise converse. Visual analog pain scales, anatomical pain depictions, and pre-established Spanish or bilingual illustrated handouts are examples of such ancillary devices. Whenever English-speaking health care providers are stumped by rehabilitation terms that must be translated into Spanish, they should consider utilizing Google España, typing the English word or phrase into the search word box, and then adding the word "Spanish." The annotated translation then usually appears below in dictionary, encyclopedic, or article format.

## DISCUSSION QUESTIONS AND ACTIVITIES

1. Select ten commonly used English language rehabilitation-related words and phrases from your practice. Find their meanings and explanations in Spanish on Google.es.

2. Take a commonly used exercise handout from your practice or that of a colleague and adapt it for Spanish-speaking patients' use.

3. Develop a time sequence continuum (*continuo*) with stick-figure drawings (*dibujos de palos*), and Spanish captions for lower

extremity swing-phase (*la fase de balancear la pierna*) gait analysis.

4. Which additional activities of daily living (*actividades de la vida cotidiana*) need to be added to the ADL list in this chapter?

5. Develop a captioned crutch-walking instruction handout for patients in Spanish.

## REFERENCES AND READINGS

1. Kendall FP, McCreary EK, Provance PG. *Muscles: Testing and function,* 4th ed. 1993, Baltimore, MD: Williams and Wilkins.

2. Como manejar y controlar el dolor de espalda en la región lumbar. 1999, San Antonio, TX: US Army Center for Health Promotion and Preventive Medicine.

3. www.bamc.amedd.army.mil/ACC [Brooke Army Medical Center's Amputee Care Center].

4. www.nlm.nih.gov/medlineplus/spanish/ency [NIH-sponsored free medical Spanish encyclopedia].

# Chapter 7

# Special Considerations

*Translators can and should provide assistance with vital English-Spanish communications between health care professionals and patients. Certain communications, including anesthesia and perioperative informed consent, require translator assistance when patients do not speak English, because of their critical importance. Spanish translators should be readily available in medical centers, hospitals, and surgical clinics. This book introduces a small selection of Spanish medical abbreviations. However, except for the Spanish abbreviations for AIDS and HIV, readers are not encouraged to use them at this point in their Spanish language acquisition. Most Spanish medical abbreviations are distinct from those in English. They do not have to be learned, in part because they are not widely known or used (except for SIDA and VIH) in the United States by the Spanish-speaking public. Readers should begin to assimilate additional verbs into their lexica. The chapter concludes with present tense conjugation of three common verbs.*

## OBJECTIVES

1. Understand the importance of medical translators for critical communications such as anesthesia and surgical consent.
2. Have available and utilize Spanish (and other language) translators when appropriate.
3. Develop formal and informal networks of translators for your clinic, facility, or system.
4. Know and appropriately use key Spanish language medical abbreviations, such as *SIDA* and *VIH*.

5. Assimilate new useful Spanish verbs in the present tense into your lexicon.

## VOCABULARY

*Las abreviaturas médicas* (medical abbreviations)

*Conducir* (to drive)

*La conjugación* (conjugation)

*Dejar* (to allow, permit, or leave)

*Los/las hispanos/as* (Hispanics)

*No se preocupe* (Don't worry)

*La pareja* (partner, significant other) [also "couple"]

*La ruta directa* (direct route)

*Venir* (to come)

# Translators Are Closer Than You May Think

Translators should be universally available to provide assistance with vital English-Spanish communications between health care professionals and patients. Certain classes of health-related communications always require translator assistance because of their critical importance. These include, but are not limited to, anesthesia, home care instructions, perioperative informed consent, and safety tips.

It may constitute a violation of accreditation standards and local, state, and federal regulatory requirements not to have translation assistance available for provider-patient care-related communications. If a Spanish-speaking patient is injured as a result of a lack of translation support, then the responsible provider(s) and facility may face health care malpractice liability exposure.

Health care providers and organizations have ample notice from demographics that a substantial number of patients and clients in the United States are Spanish speaking. The blended ethical and legal duty of effective communication requires them to utilize translators as needed, so that Spanish-speaking patients understand their health care providers and are understood by them.

As previously stated in Chapter 2, patient injury from ineffective communication is a form of professional negligence, or substandard care. Effective communication between health care providers and patients entails imparting vital care-related information that is accurate, comprehensive, timely, and mutually understood.

To establish professional negligence, a patient must prove the following elements in court: (1) that the provider owed the patient a professional duty of care; (2) that the provider violated or breached the duty owed; (3) that the violation of the standard of care caused physical and/or mental injury to the patient; and (4) that the patient is entitled to money "damages" as a result, in order to make the patient as whole again as possible. The standard (or burden) of proof for proving each of these required elements in civil malpractice trials is "preponderance of the evidence," which equates to "more likely than not" that the trier of fact (jury, or judge acting as fact-finder when there is no jury in the case) believes that the patient plaintiff's evidence presented at trial is more credible than that of the health professional-defendant.

## The Four Requisite Elements of Proof for a Patient-Plaintiff in a Professional Negligence Health Care Malpractice Trial

1. The defendant-health care provider owed the patient a special duty of due care;
2. The defendant-health care provider violated the special duty owed;
3. The patient was injured as a result; and
4. The patient is entitled to legally recognized money damages.

Besides adverse legal and ethical effects associated with ineffective patient communication—including the failure to translate when necessary—there are adverse practical consequences as well. According to Brody, patients with "limited health literacy" suffer many negative consequences, including failure to adhere to drug prescriptions, poor control of chronic conditions, overutilization of emergency rooms, and relative increased hospitalizations and mortality.[1]

Spanish translators do not necessarily have to be on-site in medical facilities in order to provide vital translation assistance, although their presence on-site constitutes optimal practice. In select practice settings in particular, such as home health and solo private practices, it may be both expedient and legally acceptable to rely on online and telephonic translation services such as www.freetranslation.com and www.languageline.com, AT&T's confidential medical translation service.

Providers can also tap into volunteer translator networks that exist in many medical centers and systems, often without cost. Examples include those translator networks at military and veterans' affairs medical centers.

# Medical Abbreviations (*Abreviaturas médicas*)– Don't Stress Over Them!

This book largely ignores Spanish medical abbreviations. Most Spanish medical abbreviations are distinct from those in English. They do not have to be learned, in part because they are not widely known or used (except for *SIDA* and *VIH*) by the Spanish-speaking public.

A sampling of Spanish language medical abbreviations includes the following:

> *AIT (ataque isquémico transitorio):* TIA (transitory ischemic attack)
>
> *EE.UU. (Estados Unidos):* USA (United States)
>
> *IMC (índice de masa corporal):* BMI (body mass index)
>
> *IU (infección urinaria):* UTI (urinary tract infection)
>
> *IV (intravenoso):* intravenous
>
> *MOR (movimiento ocular rápido):* REM (rapid eye movement)
>
> *SIDA (sindrome de inmunodeficiencia adquirida):* AIDS
>
> *TBC (tuberculosis):* TB (tuberculosis)
>
> *TC (tomografía computarizada):* CT scan
>
> *VEB (virus Epstein-Barr):* EBV (Epstein-Barr virus)
>
> *VIH (virus de inmunodeficiencia humano):* HIV

# Driving Safely to Reach Effective Communication with Hispanic Patients and Their Significant Others–Take the Easiest, Most Direct Route

Now that you have learned some of the basics of elemental Spanish, it is time for you to make the decision to continue your study of the Spanish language, most effectively through formal coursework and intensive practice and refinement of conversational skills in Spanish. The means to the end—the commitment to advance in Spanish and improved patient outcomes and satisfaction with care—makes the process well worth the effort.

Along the way, there is nothing wrong with filling in the gaps of your emerging Spanish vocabulary with English and Spanglish. Spanglish is what most limited English proficiency language learners use to communicate with non-Spanish speakers. You can and must do so, too, for now.

---

*Practice makes one more perfect, so keep up your practice of conversational Spanish!*

---

Let's end this brief final chapter on elemental Spanish with conjugation of three additional Spanish verbs in the present tense—*dejar, hacer,* and *venir.*

Normally, Spanish verbs ending in *–ar* form the present tense by dropping the *–ar* ending and adding: *o, a, amos,* or *an* to become "I _____," "you/he/she/it _____(s)," "we _____," and "you (plural)/they _____." In Chapter 4, we looked at one *–ar* verb, *estar* (to be), which does not follow this pattern exactly. Such verbs are called irregular verbs. For example, the first-person singular present tense of *estar* is *estoy* instead of *esto. Dejar* (to allow or permit, or to leave) is a regular Spanish *-ar* verb that follows the normal pattern outlined above. It is conjugated in the present tense as follows:

*Yo dejo   Usted deja   El/ella deja   Nosotros dejamos*
*Ustedes/ellas/ellos dejan*

---

*Exercise #11: Conjugate two irregular verbs, hacer (to do or make) and venir (to come), in the present tense. Use a Spanish dictionary verb table to help you.*

---

## *Hacer (to do or to make)*

| 1st sing. | 2nd sing. | 3rd sing. | 1st person plural | 2nd person plural | 3rd person plural |
|---|---|---|---|---|---|
| *Hago* | _____ | _____ | _____ | _____ | _____ |

## *Venir (to come)*

| 1st sing. | 2nd sing. | 3rd sing. | 1st person plural | 2nd person plural | 3rd person plural |
|---|---|---|---|---|---|
| *Vengo* | *Viene* | _____ | _____ | _____ | _____ |

## SUMMARY

Medical translation services are critically important in order to fulfill ethical, fiduciary, and legal duties owed to Spanish-speaking patients. Some services, especially anesthesia and perioperative care, require translation when patients and providers do not understand each other. Failure to provide medical translation services when needed may constitute professional negligence, which is a form of health care malpractice. Medical translation services are readily available to primary health care providers online, via the telephone, and in-person. Because Spanish medical abbreviations are generally utilized less often, and are not widely understood by the general public in the United States, it is recommended that readers not learn them at this time. While Spanglish and English continue to be useful for communicating with Spanish-speaking patients and for scaffolding readers' Spanish language acquisition, it is now time for you to consider formal Spanish language study in order to advance. Practice does make one more perfect, so keep it up!

## DISCUSSION QUESTIONS AND ACTIVITIES

1. Examine the online medical translation sites cited below. Evaluate their standards of medical ethics, especially concerning patient confidentiality.

2. Assume that you are a primary health care provider in private practice. How will you deal with the administrative costs associated with medical translation services?

3. What issues, if any, may arise from using patients' family members as medical translators?

4. What are some possible reasons why medical abbreviations are apparently less popular with the general public in Spanish-speaking countries than they are in the United States?

5. Conjugate the regular Spanish verb *levantar* (to raise) in the present tense.

6. Attempt to conjugate the Spanish verb *ir* (to go) in the preterite (past) tense, using a verb table from a comprehensive Spanish dictionary.

## REFERENCES AND READINGS

1. Brody J. The importance of knowing what the doctor is talking about. *New York Times.* Jan. 30, 2007, D7.

2. Brody J. To protect against drug errors, ask questions. *New York Times.* Jan. 2, 2007, D7.

3. Kaplan M. Wie sagt man…? Sites that'll translate anything. *USA Weekend.* October 8–10, 2004, 16.

4. www.freetranslation.com [medical translation assistance].

5. www.languageline.com [AT&T's confidential medical translation service].

# Epilogue: I Told You So!

In the few days or weeks since you started to read this book, you hopefully have come a long way. You have been exposed to the history, structure, grammar, and dialectal differences of the Spanish language. You have learned that a hybrid language—Spanglish—is used by millions of Spanish speakers in the United States, and can be co-opted by you to aid communication with your Spanish-speaking patients, clients, and their significant others.

From your reading, you have completed 11 exercises, including developing an elemental informed consent template in Spanish, performing two-way translation of simple dialogue, and putting together a Spanish language crutch-walking handout. You have been introduced to some 500 basic and medically focused words, phrases, and sentences in Spanish that can help you communicate with Spanish-speaking patients in your clinic.

You have learned that spoken Spanish is one of most straightforward languages to learn, principally because its vowel sounds are authentic. What you see is literally what you get.

You have learned that, like Spanish-speaking English language learners, you can use Spanglish to fill in the gaps early in your development of Spanish language competency. You have also become aware of the need to acquire and effectively use a comprehensive Spanish-language dictionary. Finally, you have realized that in order to advance as a Spanish speaker, you must do three things—relinquish Spanglish in favor of traditional Spanish, practice Spanish at least every other day, and undertake additional formal Spanish language study.

I hope that your self-confidence has grown since you have read this book. I also hope that you appreciate how important it is for you, as a clinical health care professional, to be at least elemental in conversational

Spanish in order to serve Spanish-speaking patients and clients. I also hope that you will continue to study and enjoy the Spanish language, through appropriate college course work or equivalent study.

All the best. *¡Buena suerte! Gracias por todo que ustedes hacen para sus pacientes. ¡Que Dios os bendiga!*

# Appendix A: Quick Guide

## WORDS AND PHRASES FOR SUCCESSFUL HEALTH CARE PROVIDER-HISPANIC PATIENT COMMUNICATIONS.

The following basic, key, and supportive medical Spanish words are presented first in English/Spanish word order for quick reference, then in Spanish/English word order for purposes of retention, or for use when translating a word or phrase spoken by a patient.

### English/Spanish Word Order:

A: *un, una*

Abduction: *abducción*

Abortion: *aborto voluntario*

Ache or hurt, to: *doler*

Activities: *actividades*

Adduction: *aducción*

Address: *dirección, domicilio*

Admission: *ingreso*

Adolescent: *adolescente*

Aerobic (exercise): *aeróbico*

Afternoon, late: *tarde*

Agonist: *agonista*

Aide: *asistente (la/el)*

AIDS: *SIDA (sindrome inmunodeficiencia adquirida) (el)*

Allow, permit, or to leave, to: *dejar*

Alternative: *alternativa/o*

Alternative treatments: *tratamientos alternativos*

Ambulatory: *ambulatorio*

American: *estadounidense (la/el)*

Analgesic gel: *gel analgésico*

Ankle: *tobillo*

Anorexia: *anorexia*

Antagonist: *antagonista*

Antiretroviral drugs: *antiretrovirales*

Anus: *ano*

Apart: *separado*

Appendicitis: *apendicítis*

Appointment: *cita*

Arm/arms: *brazo/brazos*

Arteries: *arterias*

Arthritis: *artritis*

Article: *artículo*

Artist: *artista (la/el)*

As soon as I/we/you/he/she/they can: *lo más pronto possible*

Asthma: *asma*

Back view: *detrás*

Backward: *hacia atrás*

Baby: *bebé (la/el)*

Balance: *equilibrio*

Be, to: *estar* [used to describe a condition, like illness]

Be, to: *ser* [used to describe identity]

Because: *porque*

Benefits: *beneficios*

Biceps: *bíceps (braquial)*

Bicycle: *bicicleta*

Big: *grande*

Bigger: *más grande*

Bipolar disorder: *trastorno bipolar*

Birth control: *control de la natalidad*

Black: *negra/o*

Blister: *ampolla*

Blonde: *rubia/o*

Blouse: *blusa*

Blue: *azul*

Body hair: *vello*

Bone: *hueso*

Book: *libro*

Boy: *niño*

Bra: *sujetador*

Brain: *cerebro*

Breast: *seno*

Breastfeed: *dar pecho*

Brown: *marrón*

Bruise: *cardenal* [also *contusión*]

Burning: *quemante*

Bus: *autobús*

Buttocks: *nalgas*

Caesarean section: *Cesárea*

Calf: *pantorrilla*

Call, to: *llamar*

Cancer: *cáncer (el)*

Car: *coche/carro*

Cardiovascular: *cardiovascular*

Cerebral vascular accident: *derrame cerebral*

Cervical: *cervical*

Cervix: *cérvix*

Chest: *pecho*

Chickenpox: *varicela*

Circulation: *circulación*

Clinic: *clínica*

Clitoris: *clítoris*

Closed chain: *cadena cerrada*

Close pack joint position: *posición cerrada*

Coat: *abrigo*

Cold pack: *compresa fría*

Collarbone: *clavícula*

Come, to: *venir*

Come in: *pase*

Communication: *comunicación*

Companion: *compañera/o*

Condom: *condón*

Conference: *conferencia* [also *congreso*]

Conjugation: *conjugación*

Constant: *constante*

Consultation: *consulta*

Coordination: *coordinación*

Crutches: *muletas*

Crutch walking: *andar con muletas*

Dark: *oscura/o*

Dark hair or skin: *morena/o*

Daughter/son: *hija/o*

December: *Diciembre*

Definite: *determinado*

Deltoids: *deltoides*

Dentist: *dentista (la/el)*

Depressed: *deprimida/o*

Depression: *depresión*

Diabetes: *diabetes*

Diagnosis: *diagnóstico*

Difficult: *difícil*

Direct access: *acceso directo*

Direct route: *ruta directa*

Dislocation: *dislocación*

Dizziness: *mareo*

Do or make, to: *hacer*

Doctor: Doctor, *doctora (el/la)*

Documentation: *documentación*

Dog, female/male: *perra/o*

Down: *abajo*

Drawing: *dibujo*
Drink, to: *beber*
Drive, to: *conducir*
Dress: *vestido*
Dry: *seca/o*
Dull: *pesado*
Dynamic strength: *fuerza dinámica*
Dyslexia: *dislexia*
Ear: *oreja*
Eardrum: *tímpano*
Early: *temprano*
Easy, facile: *fácil*
Eat, to: *comer*
Eight: *ocho*
Eighteen: *dieciocho*
Eighty: *ochenta*
Ejaculation: *eyaculación*
Elbow: *codo*
Electrical stimulation: *estimulación eléctrica*
Eleven: *once*
E-mail: *correo electrónico*
Emotional problems: *problemas emocionales*
Employee: *empleada/o*
End, closure: *final*
Erection: *erección*
European: *europea/o*
Everyday: *cotidiana*
Examine, to: *examinar*
Example: *ejemplo*
Exhale: *exhalar*
Extension: *extensión (or poner derecho)*
External: *externa*
Extremities: *extremidades*
Eye: *ojo*

Face: *cara*

Fall: *caída*

Fallopian tubes: *tubos*

Fair: *regular*

February: *febrero*

Female: *hembra*

Femur: *fémur*

Fever: *fiebre*

Fill out, to: [papers] *rellenar*

Fine: *bien*

Fifteen: *quince*

Fifty: *cincuenta*

Finger(s)/toe(s): *dedo(s)*

Five: *cinco*

Flat: *plana/o*

Foot: *pie*

Forearm: *antebrazo*

Forearm crutches: *muletas del antebrazo*

Forty: *cuarenta*

Forward: *adelante*

Four: *cuatro*

Fourteen: *catorce*

Flexion: *flexión (or doblar)*

Fracture: *fractura*

Friday: *Viernes*

Front view: *de frente*

Gall bladder: *vesícula biliar*

Gastrocnemius: *gastrocnemio*

Get up, to: *levantarse*

Girl: *niña*

Give birth: *dar luz*

Go, to: *ir*

Goals: *metas*

Good: *buena/o*

Good afternoon: *buenas tardes*
Goodbye: *adiós*
Good evening/good night: *buenas noches*
Good morning: *buenos dias*
Grandchild: *nieta/o*
Gray: *gris*
Green: *verde*
Gums: *encías*
Hair on one's head: *cabello*
Hand: *mano (la)*
Happy: *feliz*
Hard: *dura/o*
Have, to: *tener*
He, they: *él, ellos*
Head: *cabeza*
Health record: *historial médico*
Heart: *corazón*
Heavy build: *gorda/o*
Height: *altura*
Hepatitis: *hepatitis*
Hi: *hola*
High/tall: *alta/o*
High blood pressure: *tensión alta*
High cholesterol: *colesterol elevado*
Hip: *cadera*
Hispanics: *hispanos*
HIV: *VIH (virus de inmunodeficiencia humano) (el)*
Home exercises: *ejercicios para casa*
Hot pack: *compresa caliente*
Hour, time: *hora*
House: *casa*
How are you? *¿Cómo está?*
How do you say….? *¿Cómo se dice…?*
How long? *¿Cuánto tiempo?*

How many/much? *¿Cuánto?*

Humerus: *humero*

Hurt, to: *doler*

I: *yo*

Ice: *hielo*

Ilium: *hueso ilíaco*

Ill: *enferma/o*

I'm sorry: *Lo siento*

Immunization: *vacunación*

Indefinite: *indeterminado*

Infection: *infección*

Informed consent: *consentimiento informado*

Inhale: *inspirar*

Injection: *inyección*

Inpatient: *paciente hospitalizado*

Inside: *adentro*

Intensity: *intensidad*

Intensive care: *terapia intensiva*

Intercostals: *intercostales*

Intermittent: *me va y me viene*

Internal: *interna*

Isometric: *isométrica*

Isotonic: *isotónica*

January: *enero*

Jaw: *mandíbula*

July: *julio*

June: *junio*

Kidneys: *riñones*

Knee: *rodilla*

Kyphosis: *cifosis*

Lab test: *análisis de laboratorio*

Labor pains: *dolores del parto*

Laceration: *laceración*

Large: *grande*

Large intestine: *intestino grueso*
Left: *izquierda/o*
Leg: *pierna*
Length: *longitud*
Lengthening: *alargamiento*
Less: *menos*
Letter: *carta*
Light (color): *clara/o*
Light: *luz*
Limp: *cojera*
Lips: *labios*
Liver: *hígado*
Local: *local*
Long (height): *larga/o*
Lordosis: *lordosis*
Low, short (height): *baja/o*
Low back pain: *dolor de espalda*
Lower, to: *bajar*
Lumbar: *lumbar*
Lungs: *pulmones*
Male: *macho*
Mammogram: *mamograma*
Managed care: *medicina gerenciada*
Manic: *maníaca/o*
Manipulation: *manipulación*
March: *marzo*
Married: *casada/o*
Massage: *masaje*
Mastectomy: *mastectomía*
Material risks: *riesgos importantes*
May: *mayo*
Measles: *sarampión*
Medical abbreviations: *abreviaturas médicas*
Medical insurance: *seguro médico*

Medication: *medicación, medicamento*
Medicine: *medicina*
Menopause: *menopausia*
Menstrual cycle: *ciclo menstrual*
Menstruation: *menstruación*
Mild: *leve*
Mine: *mío*
Minute: *minuto*
Miscarriage: *aborto involuntario*
Mobility: *movilidad*
Mobilization: *movilización*
Model: *modelo (la/el)*
Moderate: *moderado*
Mole, surface of the moon: *lunar*
Monday: *lunes*
More: *más*
Morning, tomorrow: *mañana*
Mouth: *boca*
Move, to: *mover*
Mr., Mrs., Ms.: *Señor, Señora, Señorita*
Mumps: *paperas*
Muscle fatigue: *fatiga muscular*
Muscular contraction: *contracción muscular*
My, singular/plural: *mi, mis*
Myocardial infarction: *infarto de miocardio*
Nausea: *nausea*
Navel: *ombligo*
Need, to: *necesitar*
No: *no*
Neck: *cuello*
Nervous: *nerviosa/o*
Neurosis: *neurosis*
Night: *noche*
Nine: *nueve*

Nineteen: *diecinueve*

Ninety: *noventa*

Nipple: *pezón*

Normal: *normal*

Nose: *nariz*

Nothing: *nada*

November: *Noviembre*

Nuclear family: *familia nuclear*

Numb, to feel: *sentir dormido*

Nurse, female/male: *enfermera, enfermero*

Obsessive-compulsive disorder: *trastorno obsesivocompulsivo*

Occupational therapist: *terapeuta ocupacional (la/el)*

October: *octubre*

Office: *oficina*

Oil (on skin): *grasa/o*

On foot: *a pie*

One: *uno*

One hundred: *cien*

One thousand: *mil*

Open chain: *cadena abierta*

Open pack joint position: *posición abierta*

Operating room team: *equipo quirúrgico*

Orgasm: *orgasmo*

Ours: *nuestra/o*

Outpatient: *paciente ambulatorio*

Outside: *afuera*

Pain: *dolor*

Pain scale: *escala del dolor*

Pancreas: *páncreas*

Pants: *pantalones*

Paper: *papel*

Pap smear: *examen Papanicolau (el Pap)*

Paraffin: *parafina*

Pardon Me: *Perdóneme*

Partner, significant other [also "couple"]: *pareja*

Patella: *rótula*

Patient: *paciente (la/el)*

Patient care: *atención al paciente/a la paciente*

Patient instructions: *instrucciones al paciente*

Pectoralis Major: *pectoral mayor*

Pelvis: *pelvis*

Pen: *boligrafo*

Pencil: *lápiz*

Penis: *pene*

Pediatric: *pediatra*

Period: *período/regla*

Perioperative care: *atencion quirurgico*

Phalanges (hands and feet): *falanges*

Phase: *fase*

Physical therapist: *terapeuta fisica (la/el)*

Pink: *rosado*

Please: *por favor*

Please remove your….: *Quítese por favor su….*

Plumb line: *línea recta a plomo*

Point (with a finger): *apunte*

Pregnant: *embarazada/encinta*

Pregnancy: *embarazo*

Prescription: *receta*

Problem: *problema (el)*

Prognosis: *prognóstico*

Prostate: *próstata*

Psychiatric problems: *problemas psiquiátricos*

Psychosis: *psicosis*

Push: *aprete*

Quadriceps: *cuádriceps*

Questions: *preguntas*

Quickly: *rápidamente*

Radiating: *extendido*

Radius: *radio*
Raise, to: *levantar*
Raised: *elevada/o*
Receptionist: *recepcionista (la/el)*
Rectus Abdominus: *recto del abdomen*
Red: *rojo*
Red-headed: *pelirroja/o*
Referral: *recomendación*
Referral order: *volante*
Rehabilitation team: *equipo de rehabilitación*
Relax, to: *relajar*
Repeat, to: *repetir*
Repetitions: *repeticiones*
Research study: *investigación*
Research subject: *participante (la/el)*
Resistance, endurance: *resistencia*
Rib: *costilla*
Right: *derecha/o*
Robe: *bata*
Room: *cuarto*
Rotation: *rotación*
Rough: *áspera/o*
Sad: *triste*
Saturday: *sábado*
Scapula: *omóplato* [also *escápula*]
Schizoprenia: *esquizofrenia*
Scoliosis: *escoliosis*
Seat: *asiento*
Second: *segundo* [unit of time and ordinal number]
Semen: *semen*
September: *septiembre*
Seven: *siete*
Seventeen: *diecisiete*
Seventy: *setenta*

Severe: *severo*
Sharp: *agudo*
She, they: *ella, ellas*
Shin: *espinilla*
Shirt: *camisa*
Shoes: *zapatos*
Shoulder: *hombro*
Show me: *Enséñeme*
Sit down, to: *sentarse*
Six: *seis*
Sixteen: *dieciseis* [10 + 6]
Sixty: *sesenta*
Skeletal muscle: *músculo esquelético*
Skirt: *falda*
Skull: *cráneo*
Slowly: *lentamente*
Small: *pequeña/o*
Small intestine: *intestino delgado*
Smaller: *más pequena/o*
Smooth: *suave*
Socks: *calcetines*
Some: *unos, unas*
Sort (length): *corta/o*
Spanish: *Español*
Speed: *velocidad*
Spleen: *bazo*
Spouse: *esposa/o*
Stabilizer (muscle): *estabilizador*
Static strength: *fuerza estática*
Steps: *pasos*
Sternocleidomastoid: *esternocleidomastoideo*
Sternum: *esternón*
Sticks: *palos*
Stomach: *estómago*

Straight: *recto*

Strength: *fuerza*

Strengthen, to: *fortalecer*

Stretch, to: *estirar*

Striated muscle: *músculo estriado*

Sunday: *domingo*

Symptoms: *síntomas*

Synergist: *sinergista*

Take, to: *tomar*

Talk: *hablar*

The: *el, la, las, lo, los*

Teacher: *profesor, profesora*

Ten: *diez*

Testicles: *testículos*

Thanks: *gracias*

That's enough: *Ya está*

Therapy: *terapia (la)*

Therapy pool: *piscina terapéutica*

There is…: *Hay…*

Thigh: *muslo*

Thin build: *delgada/o*

Thirteen: *trece*

Thirty: *treinta*

This one: *ésta/e/o*

Three: *tres*

Throat: *garganta*

Thumb(s): *pulgar(es)*

Thursday: *jueves*

Tie, to: *atar*

Time, as in "one time": *vez ("una vez")*

Tingling sensation: *cosquillas/hormigueo*

Today: *hoy*

Toddler: *niña pequeña/niño pequeño*

Together: *junto(s)*

Tongue: *lengua*

Tooth/teeth: *diente(s)*

Trace: *vestigio*

Traction: *tracción*

Transcutaneous electrical nerve stimulation: *estímulo eléctrico transcutáneo del nervio*

Translation: *traducción*

Translator: *traductor/a*

Trapezius: *trapezio*

Treadmill: *rueda de ardilla* [literally "squirrel wheel"]

Treatment: *tratamiento médico*

Triceps: *tríceps*

Trunk: *tronco*

Tuberculosis: *tuberculosis*

Tuesday: *martes*

Twelve: *doce*

Twenty: *veinte*

Two: *dos*

Ulna: *cúbito*

Ultrasound: *ultrasonido*

Until tomorrow/the next appointment: *Hasta mañana/la próxima visita.*

Up: *arriba*

Urethra: *uretra*

Urinary bladder: *vejiga*

Uterus: *utero*

Vagina: *vagina*

Vaginal discharge: *secreción vaginal*

Vasectomy: *vasectomía*

Veins: *venas*

Vertebral column: *columna vertebral*

Vocabulary: *vocabulario*

Volume: *volúmen*

Vomiting: *vómitos*

Waist: *cintura*

Walk, to: *andar* [also *caminar*]

Walker: *andador (el)*

Water: *agua (el)* [but *las aguas* plural]

We: *nosotros*

Weak: *débil*

Wednesday: *miércoles*

Week: *semana*

Weight: *peso*

Weightbearing: *peso sobre la pierna débil*

Weightlifting: *levantamiento de pesas*

Weights: *pesas*

Welcome: *bienvenido*

Wet: *mojada/o*

Wheelchair: *silla de ruedas*

When? *¿Cuándo?*

Where? *¿Donde?*

Whirlpool bath: *baño de remolino*

White: *blanco*

Why? *¿Por que?*

Wide: *ancha/o*

Wrist: *muñeca*

Wrist bones: *carpos*

Work, to: *trabajar*

Worry about, to: *preocuparse*

X-ray: *radiografía*

Yellow: *amarillo*

Yes, if: *sí*

Yesterday: *ayer*

You, familiar, singular [Use with a child patient.]: *tú*

You, formal, singular: *usted*

You, formal, plural: *ustedes*

You are welcome: *de nada*

Your, their, yours, theirs: *su, sus*

Zero: *cero*

**Spanish/English word order:**

*Abajo:* down

*Abducción:* abduction

*Aborto involuntario:* miscarriage

*Aborto voluntario:* abortion

*Abreviaturas médicas:* medical abbreviations

*Abrigo:* coat

*Acceso directo:* direct access

*Actividades:* activities

*Adelante:* forward

*Adentro:* inside

*Adiós:* Goodbye

*Adolescente:* adolescent

*Aducción:* adduction

*Aeróbico:* aerobic (exercise)

*Afuera:* outside

*Agonista:* agonist

*Agua (el):* water

*Agudo:* sharp

*Alargamiento:* lengthening

*Alta/o:* high, tall

*Alternativa/o:* alternative

*Altura:* height

*Amarillo:* yellow

*Ambulatorio:* ambulatory

*Ampolla:* blister

*Análisis de laboratorio:* lab test

*Ancha/o:* wide

*Andador:* walker

*Andar:* to walk [also caminar]

*Andar con muletas:* crutch walking

*Ano:* anus

*Anorexia:* anorexia

*Antagonista:* antagonist

*Antebrazo:* forearm

*Antiretrovirales:* antiretroviral drugs

*Apendicítis:* appendicitis

*A pie:* on foot

*Aprete:* push

*Apunte:* point (with a finger)

*Arriba:* up

*Arterias:* arteries

*Articulo:* article

*Artista (la/el):* artist

*Artritis:* arthritis

*Asiento:* seat

*Asistente (la/el):* aide

*Asma:* asthma

*Áspera/o:* rough

*Atar:* to tie

*Atención al paciente/a la paciente:* patient care

*Atención quirúrgico:* perioperative care

*Autobús:* by bus

*Ayer:* yesterday

*Azul:* blue

*Bajar:* to lower

*Baja/o:* low, short (height)

*Baño de remolino:* whirlpool bath

*Bata:* robe

*Bazo:* spleen

*Bebé (la/el):* baby

*Beber:* to drink

*Beneficios:* benefits

*Bíceps (braquial):* Biceps

*Bicicleta:* bicycle

*Bien:* fine

*Bienvenido:* Welcome

*Blanco:* white

*Blusa:* blouse

*Boca:* mouth

*Bolígrafo:* pen

*Brazo/brazos:* arm/arms

*Buena:* good

*Buenos días:* Good morning

*Buenas tardes:* Good afternoon

*Buenas noches:* Good evening/good night

*Cabello:* hair on one's head

*Cabeza:* head

*Cadena abierta:* open chain

*Cadena cerrada:* closed chain

*Cadera:* hip

*Caída:* fall

*Calcetines:* socks

*Camisa:* shirt

*Cáncer (el):* cancer

*Cara:* face

*Cardenal:* bruise [also la contusión]

*Cardiovascular:* cardiovascular

*Carpos:* wrist bones

*Carta:* letter

*Casa:* house

*Casada/o:* married

*Catorce:* fourteen

*Cerebro:* brain

*Cervical:* cervical

*Cesárea:* Caesarean section

*Cero:* zero

*Cérvix:* cervix

*Ciclo menstrual:* menstrual cycle

*Cien:* one hundred

*Cifosis:* kyphosis

*Cinco:* five

*Cincuenta:* fifty

*Cintura:* waist

*Circulación:* circulation

*Cita:* appointment

*Clara/o:* light

*Clavícula:* collarbone

*Clínica:* clinic

*Clítoris:* clitoris

*Coche/carro:* car

*Codo:* elbow

*Cojera:* limp

*Colesterol elevado:* high cholesterol

*Columna vertebral:* vertebral column

*Comer:* to eat

*¿Cómo está?* How are you?

*¿Cómo se dice...?* How do you say...?

*Compañera/o:* companion

*Compresa caliente:* hot pack

*Compresa fría:* cold pack

*Comunicación:* communication

*Condón:* condom

*Conducir:* to drive

*Conferencia:* conference [also congreso]

*Conjugación:* conjugation

*Consentimiento informado:* informed consent

*Constante:* constant

*Consulta:* consultation

*Contracción muscular:* muscle contraction

*Control de la natalidad:* birth control

*Coordinación:* coordination

*Corazón:* heart

*Correo electrónico:* e-mail

*Corta/o:* short (length)

*Cosquillas/hormigueo:* tingling sensation

*Costilla:* rib

*Cotidiana:* everyday

*Cráneo:* skull

*Cuádriceps:* quadriceps

*¿Cuándo?* When?

*¿Cuánto?* How many/much?

*¿Cuánto tiempo?* How long?

*Cúbito:* ulna

*Cuarenta:* forty

*Cuarto:* room

*Cuatro:* four

*Cuello:* neck

*Dar luz:* give birth

*Dar pecho:* breastfeed

*Débil:* weak

*Dedo(s):* finger(s), toe(s)

*De frente:* front view

*Dejar:* to allow, permit, or to leave

*Delgada/o:* thin build

*Deltoides:* deltoids

*De nada:* You're welcome

*Dentista (la/el):* dentist

*Depresión:* depression

*Deprimida/o:* depressed

*Derecha/o:* right

*Derrame cerebral:* cerebral vascular accident

*Desorden de deficiencia de atención debido a la hiperactividad:* attention deficit hyperactivity disorder

*Determinado:* definite

*Detrás:* back view

*Diabetes:* diabetes

*Diagnóstico:* diagnosis

*Dibujo:* drawing

*Diciembre:* December

*Dieciseis:* sixteen [10 + 6]

*Diecisiete:* seventeen

*Dieciocho:* eighteen

*Diecinueve:* nineteen

*Diente(s):* tooth, teeth

*Diez:* ten

*Difícil:* difficult

*Dirección, domicilio:* address

*Dislexia:* dyslexia

*Dislocación:* dislocation

*Doce:* twelve

*Doctor, doctora:* Dr.

*Documentación:* documentation

*Doler:* to ache or hurt

*Dolor:* pain

*Dolor de espalda:* low back pain

*Dolores del parto:* labor pains

*Domingo:* Sunday

*Donde:* where

*Dos:* two

*Dura/o:* hard

*Ejemplo:* example

*Ejercicios para casa:* home exercises

*El, la, las, lo, los:* the

*Él, ellos:* he, they

*Ella, ellas:* she, they

*Embarazada/encinta:* pregnant

*Embarazo:* pregnancy

*Empleada/o:* employee

*Encías:* gums

*Enero:* January

*Enferma:* ill

*Enfermera, enfermero:* nurse female/male

*Enséñeme:* Show me

*Equilibrio:* balance

*Equipo quirúrgico:* operating room team

*Equipo de rehabilitación:* rehabilitation team

*Erección:* erection

*Escala del dolor:* pain scale

*Escoliosis:* scoliosis

*Español:* Spanish

*Espinilla:* shin

*Esposa/o:* spouse

*Esquizofrenia:* schizoprenia

*Ésta/e:* this one

*Estabilizador:* stabilizer (muscle)

*Estadounidense (la/el):* American

*Estar:* to be

*Esternocleidomastoideo:* sternocleidomastoidus

*Esternón:* sternum

*Estimulación eléctrica:* electrical stimulation

*Estímulo eléctrico transcutáneo del nervio:* transcutaneous electrical nerve stimulation

*Estirar:* to stretch

*Estómago:* stomach

*Europeo/a:* European

*Examen Papanicolau (el Pap):* Pap smear

*Examinar:* to examine

*Exhalar:* exhale

*Externa:* external

*Extendido:* radiating

*Extensión (or poner derecho):* extension

*Extremidades:* extremities

*Eyaculación:* ejaculation

*Fácil:* facile

*Falanges:* phalanges (hands and feet)

*Falda:* skirt

*Familia nuclear:* nuclear family

*Fase:* phase

*Fatiga muscular:* muscle fatigue

*Febrero:* February

*Feliz:* happy

*Fémur:* femur

*Fiebre:* fever

*Final:* closure

*Flexión (or doblar):* flexion

*Fortalecer:* to strengthen

*Fractura:* fracture

*Fuerza:* strength

*Fuerza dinámica:* dynamic strength

*Fuerza estática:* static strength

*Garganta:* throat

*Gastrocnemio:* Gastrocnemius

*Gel analgésico:* analgesic gel

*Glaucoma:* glaucoma

*Gluteo mayor:* gluteus maximus

*Gorda/o:* heavy build

*Gracias:* Thanks

*Grande:* big

*Grasa/o:* oil (on skin)

*Gris:* gray

*Hablar:* to talk

*Hacer:* to do or to make

*Hacia atrás:* backward

*Hasta mañana/la próxima visita:* Until tomorrow/the next appointment.

*Hay:* There is…

*Hembra:* female

*Hepatitis:* hepatitis

*Hielo:* ice

*Hígado:* liver

*Hija/o:* daughter/son

*Hispanos:* Hispanics

*Historial medico:* health record

*Hola:* Hi

*Hombro:* shoulder

*Hora:* hour, time

*Hoy:* today

*Hueso:* bone

*Hueso ilíaco:* ilium

*Humero:* humerus

*Indeterminado:* indefinite

*Infarto de miocardio:* myocardial infarction

*Infección:* infection

*Ingreso:* admission

*Inspirar:* inhale

*Instrucciones al paciente:* patient instructions

*Intensidad:* intensity

*Intercostales:* Intercostals

*Interna:* internal

*Intestino delgado:* small intestine

*Intestino grueso:* large intestine

*Investigación:* research study

*Inyección:* injection

*Ir:* to go

*Isométrica:* isometric

*Isotónica:* isotonic

*Izquierda/o:* left

*Jueves:* Thursday

*Julio:* July

*Junio:* June

*Junto:* together

*Labios:* lips

*Laceración:* laceration

*Lápiz:* pencil

*Larga/o:* long (height)

*Lengua:* tongue
*Lentamente:* slowly
*Levantamiento de pesas:* weightlifting
*Levantar:* to raise
*Levantarse:* to get up
*Leve:* mild
*Libro:* book
*Línea recta a plomo:* plumb line
*Llamar:* to call
*Local:* local
*Lo más pronto possible*: as soon as I/we can
*Longitud:* length
*Lordosis:* lordosis
*Lo siento:* I'm sorry
*Lumbar:* lumbar
*Lunar:* mole, surface of the moon
*Lunes:* Monday
*Mamograma:* mammogram
*Macho:* male
*Mañana:* morning, tomorrow
*Mandíbula:* jaw
*Maníaca/o:* manic
*Manipulación:* manipulation
*Marrón:* brown
*Más:* more
*Masaje:* massage
*Más grande:* bigger
*Más pequeno:* smaller
*Mastectomía:* mastectomy
*Medicación, medicamento:* medication
*Medicina:* medicine
*Medicina gerenciada:* managed care
*Menopausia:* menopause
*Menos:* less

*Menstruación:* menstruation

*Metas:* goals

*Mi, mis:* my, singular, plural

*Mío/a:* mine

*Modelo (la/el):* model

*Mover:* to move

*Movilidad:* mobility

*Movilización:* mobilization

*Muletas:* crutches

*Muletas axilares:* auxiliary crutches

*Muletas del antebrazo:* forearm crutches

*Muñeca:* wrist

*Mano:* hand

*Mareo:* dizziness

*Martes:* Tuesday

*Marzo:* March

*Mayo:* May

*Me va y me viene:* intermittent

*Miércoles:* Wednesday

*Mil:* one thousand

*Minuto:* minute

*Moderado:* moderate

*Mojada/o:* wet

*Morena/o:* dark-haired

*Músculo esquelético:* skeletal muscle

*Músculo estriado:* striated muscle

*Muslo:* thigh

*Nada:* nothing

*Nariz:* nose

*Nausea:* nausea

*Necesitar:* to need

*Negro:* black

*Nerviosa/o:* nervous

*Neuropraxia axilar:* auxiliary nerve damage

*Neurosis:* neurosis
*Nieta/o:* grandchild
*Niña (la), niño (el):* girl, boy
*Niña pequeña/niño pequeño:* toddler
*No*: no
*Noche:* night
*Normal:* normal
*Nosotros:* we
*Noventa:* ninety
*Noviembre:* November
*Nuestra/o:* ours
*Nueve:* nine
*Ochenta:* eighty
*Ocho:* eight
*Octubre:* October
*Oficina:* office
*Ojo:* eye
*Ombligo:* navel
*Omóplato:* scapula [also *escápula*]
*Once*: eleven
*Oreja:* ear
*Orgasmo:* orgasm
*Oscura/o:* dark
*Paciente (la/el):* patient
*Paciente ambulatorio:* outpatient
*Paciente hospitalizado:* inpatient
*Palos:* sticks
*Páncreas*: pancreas
*Pantalones:* pants
*Pantorrilla:* calf
*Papel:* paper
*Paperas:* mumps
*Parafina:* paraffin
*Pareja:* partner, significant other [also "couple"]

*Participante (la/el):* research subject
*Pase:* Come in
*Pasos:* steps
*Pecho:* chest
*Pectoral mayor:* pectoralis major
*Pediatra:* pediatric
*Pelirroja/o:* red-head
*Pelvis:* pelvis
*Pene:* penis
*Pequeña/o:* small
*Perdóneme:* Pardon me
*Período/regla:* period
*Perra/o:* female/male dog
*Pesado:* dull
*Pesa/o:* weight
*Pesas:* weights
*Peso sobre la pierna débil:* weightbearing
*Pezón:* nipple
*Pie:* foot
*Pierna:* leg
*Piscina terapéutica:* therapy pool
*Plan/ao:* flat
*Por favor:* please
*¿Por qué?* Why?
*Porque:* because
*Posición abierta:* open pack (joint) position
*Posición cerrada:* close pack (joint) position
*Preguntas:* questions
*Preocuparse:* to worry about
*Problema (el):* problem
*Problemas emocionales:* emotional problems
*Problemas psiquiátricos:* psychiatric problems
*Profesor, profesora:* teacher
*Prognóstico:* prognosis

*Próstata:* prostate

*Psicosis:* psychosis

*Pulgar(es):* thumb(s)

*Pulmones:* lungs

*Quemante:* burning

*Quince:* fifteen

*Quítese por favor su....* Please remove your....

*Radio:* radius

*Radiografía:* x-ray

*Rápidamente:* quickly

*Recepcionista (la/el):* receptionist

*Receta:* prescription

*Recomendación:* referral

*Recto:* straight

*Recto del abdomen:* Rectus abdominus

*Regular:* fair

*Relajar:* to relax

*Rellenar:* to fill out [papers]

*Repeticiones:* repetitions

*Repetir:* to repeat

*Resistencia:* endurance, resistance

*Riesgos importantes (los):* material risks

*Riñones:* kidneys

*Rodilla:* knee

*Rojo:* red

*Rosado:* pink

*Rotación:* rotation

*Rótula:* patella

*Rubia/o:* blonde

*Rueda de ardilla:* treadmill [literally "squirrel wheel"]

*Ruta directa:* direct route

*Sábado:* Saturday

*Sarampión:* measles

*Secreción vaginal:* vaginal discharge

*Seca/o:* dry

*Segundo:* second [unit of time and ordinal number]

*Seguro medico:* medical insurance

*Seis:* six

*Semana:* week

*Semen:* semen

*Seno:* breast

*Señor, Señora, Señorita:* Mr., Mrs., Ms.

*Sentarse:* to sit down

*Sentir dormido:* to feel numb

*Separado:* apart

*Septiembre:* September

*Ser:* to be

*Sesenta:* sixty

*Setenta:* seventy

*Severo:* severe

*Sí, si:* yes, if

*SIDA (sindrome inmunodeficiencia adquirida) (el):* AIDS

*Siete:* seven

*Silla de ruedas:* wheelchair

*Sinergista:* synergist

*Síntomas*: symptoms

*Su, sus:* your, their, yours, theirs

*Sujetador:* bra

*Suave:* smooth

*Tarde:* afternoon, late

*Temprano:* early

*Tener:* to have

*Tensión alta:* high blood pressure

*Terapeuta ocupacional (la/el):* occupational therapist

*Terapeuta física (la/el):* physical therapist

*Terapia:* therapy

*Terapia intensiva:* intensive care

*Testículos:* testicles

*Tímpano:* eardrum
*Tobillo:* ankle
*Tomar:* to take
*Trabajar:* to work
*Tracción:* traction
*Traducción:* translation
*Traductor/a:* translator
*Trapezio:* Trapezius
*Trastorno bipolar:* bipolar disorder
*Trastorno obsesivocompulsivo:* obsessive-compulsive disorder
*Tratamientos alternativos:* alternative treatments
*Tratamiento médico:* treatment
*Trece:* thirteen
*Treinta:* thirty
*Tres:* three
*Tríceps:* Triceps
*Triste:* sad
*Tronco:* trunk
*Tú:* you, familiar, singular [Use with a child patient.]
*Tuberculosis:* tuberculosis
*Tubos:* Fallopian tubes
*Ultrasonido:* ultrasound
*Un, una:* a
*Uno:* one
*Unos, unas:* some
*Uretra:* urethra
*Usted:* you, formal, singular
*Ustedes:* you, formal, plural
*Utero:* uterus
*Vacunación:* immunization
*Vagina:* vagina
*Varicela:* chickenpox
*Vasectomía:* vasectomy
*Veinte:* twenty

*Vejiga:* urinary bladder

*Velocidad:* speed

*Venas:* veins

*Venir:* to come

*Verde:* green

*Vesícula biliar:* gallbladder

*Vestido:* dress

*Vestigio:* trace

*Vez:* time, as in *una vez,* "one time"

*Viernes:* Friday

*VIH (virus de inmunodeficiencia humano) (el):* HIV

*Vocabulario:* vocabulary

*Volante:* referral order

*Volúmen:* volume

*Vómitos:* vomiting

*Ya está:* That's enough

*Yo:* I

*Zapatos:* shoes

# Appendix B-1

### Patients' Rights and Responsibilities
### Brooke Army Medical Center

**We at Brooke Army Medical Center (BAMC)** hold the welfare and safety of the patient as our highest priority. The most important person in this medical center is you, our patient. Our goal is to provide you with the best medical care available. Our success will be reflected in your satisfaction with the treatment you receive. We regard your basic human rights with great importance. You have the right to freedom of expression, to make your own decisions, and to know that your human rights will be preserved and respected. The following is a list of patient rights and responsibilities.

## Your Rights as a Patient

## You have the right to receive respectful, considerate, and supportive treatment and service.

We will do our best to provide you with compassionate and respectful care at all times. We will do everything possible to provide a safe hospital environment. We will be attentive to your specific needs and requests, understanding that they should not interfere with medical care for you or for others. We will not discriminate in providing you with care, based on race, ethnicity, national origin, religion, gender, age, mental or physical disability, genetic information, sexual orientation, or source of payment.

## You have the right to be involved in all aspects of your care.

We will make sure that you know which physician or care provider is primarily responsible for your care. We will explain the professional status and the role of persons who help in your care. We will keep you fully informed about your condition, the results of tests we perform, and the treatment you receive. We will clearly explain to you any treatments or procedures that we propose. We will request your written consent for procedures that carry more than minimal risk. We will make sure that you are part of the decision-making process in your care. When there are dilemmas or differences over care decisions, we will include you in resolving them. We will honor your right to refuse the care that we advise. (In some circumstances, especially for active duty patients, laws and regulations may override this right.) We will honor your Advance Directive or Medical Power of Attorney regarding limits to the care that you wish to receive.

## You have the right to receive timely and appropriate assessment and management of your pain.

We will routinely ask if you are suffering pain. If you are, we will evaluate it further and help you get relief.

## You have the right to have your personal needs respected.

We will respect the confidentiality of your personal information throughout the institution. (For active duty persons, complete confidentiality may not be possible, based on requirements to report some conditions or findings.) We will respect your need for privacy in conversations, examinations, information sharing, and procedures. Also, you may request that a chaperone be present during an examination or procedure. We will communicate with you in a language that you understand. We will respect your need to feel safe and secure through-out the facility. Hospital employees will be identifiable with badges or nameplates. We will take your concerns and complaints seriously and will work hard to resolve them. We will respect your need for pastoral care and other spiritual services. Our Chaplain Service is on call at all times. Other spiritual support is welcome, as long as it does not inter-fere with patient care or hospital function. We will respect your need to communicate with others, both family and friends. If it is medically necessary to limit your communications with others, we will tell you and your family why. We will use soft fabric restraints, with close and frequent monitoring, if you become so confused that you are in danger of hurting yourself or others. We will untie the restraints as soon as we safely can do so.

## You have the right to receive information on how to contact protective services.

At your request, we will give you information on how you may contact protective services for children, adults, or the elderly. We will do this confidentially.

## You have the right to participate in clinical research when it is appropriate.

Your care provider will discuss this with you when it is appropriate. The Institutional Review Board, a committee that includes people from many parts of this community, monitors all research at BAMC. We will thoroughly explain the proposed research to you and ask your written permission to take part. If you choose not to take part in the research, it will not affect the care that we give you. Participation is completely voluntary.

## You have the right to speak to a BAMC Patient Representative regarding any aspect of your care.

We encourage patients and families to speak directly with ward of clinic personnel if there is a problem. However, if these people cannot solve it, you may contact the Patient Representative at 210-916-2330 (clinics) or 210-916-2200 (inpatient tower).

## You have the right to expect that this institution will operate according to a code of ethical behavior.

The Command at BAMC is firmly committed to managing this hospital according to the highest traditions of military and medical professionalism and ethics. In addition, our Institutional Bioethics Committee meets regularly to review ethical topics, including organizational ethics. This committee is available to you and to our employees if a serious ethical dilemma comes up in either patient care or service.

## You have a right to receive a personal copy of these patient rights.

Copies of these patient rights are available on any ward and in any clinic at BAMC. If you cannot locate a copy for yourself, ask ward or clinic personnel. If you have any questions or comments regarding patient rights, we encourage you to contact a BAMC Patient Representative at 210-916-2330 or 210-916-2200.

# Your Responsibilities as a Patient

You are responsible for maximizing your own healthy behaviors. You are responsible for taking an active part in decisions about your health care. You are responsible for providing us with accurate and complete information about your health and your condition. You are responsible for showing courtesy and respect for other patients, families, hospital staff, and visitors. This includes personal and hospital property. You are responsible for keeping your scheduled appointments on time, and for giving us advance notice if you must cancel or reschedule. You are responsible for providing us with your current address and means of contact (such as a home phone or cell phone). You are responsible for providing us with current information regarding any other health insurance coverage you have. You are responsible for keeping yourself informed of the coverage, options, and policies of the TRICARE plan that you subscribe to as a military beneficiary. This information is available in the TRICARE Service Office (Beneficiary Line: 1-800-406-2832).

# Appendix B-2

### Derechos y responsabilidades de los pacientes (al 19 de septiembre de 2005)

En Brooke Army Medical Center (BAMC) consideramos que el bienestar y seguridad del paciente es nuestra mayor prioridad. La persona más importante en este centro médico es usted, nuestro paciente. Nuestro objetivo es brindarle la mayor atención medica disponible. Nuestro éxito se verá reflejado en su satisfacción con el tratamiento que recibe. Le damos una gran importancia a sus derechos humanos básicos. Usted tiene derecho a tomar sus propias decisiones y a saber que sus derechos humanos serán preservados y respetados. La siguiente es una lista de derechos y responsabilidades de los pacientes.

## Sus derechos como paciente

Usted tiene el derecho a recibir un tratamiento y servicio respetuoso, considerado y sustentador. Daremos lo mejor de nosotros para brindarle una atención respetuosa y compasiva en todo momento. Haremos todo lo posible para brindarle un ambiente hospitalario seguro. Usted es responsable de mantenerse informado de la cobertura, opciones y políticas del plan TRICARE a que usted suscribe como beneficiario militario. Esta información se encuentra disponible en la Oficina de Servicios de TRICARE (Línea para beneficiarios: 1-800-406-2832).

No discriminaremos para brindarle la atención de la mejor calidad posible en función de: su capacidad de pagar su factura hospitalaria, posición económica, raza, etnia, origen nacional, religión, género, edad, incapacidad física o mental, información genética, orientación sexual o fuente de pago. El acceso a las clínicas ambulatorias es de conformidad con las normas de TRICARE.

Usted tiene el derecho a involucrarse en todos los aspectos de su atención. Nos aseguramos de que sepa qué médico o proveedor de atención es principalmente responsable por su atención. Explicaremos la posición profesional y el rol de las personas que ayudan en su atención. Lo mantendremos totalmente informado de su estado. Le explicaremos claramente todos los tratamientos o procedimientos que propongamos. Nos aseguraremos de que usted participe en el proceso de toma de decisiones sobre su atención. Cuando haya dilemas o diferencias en las decisiones sobre su atención, lo incluiremos a usted para resolverlas.

Con su permiso, involucraremos a su familia en las decisiones acerca de su atención médica. Solicitaremos su consentimiento por escrito para los procedimientos que implican más que un riesgo mínimo. Respetaremos su derecho a rechazar la atención que aconsejamos. En algunas circunstancias, especialmente para los pacientes en servicio activo, las leyes y reglamentos pueden anular este derecho. Respetaremos su Directiva Anticipada con respecto a los límites para la atención que usted desea recibir, de conformidad con la Ley de Texas. Respetaremos su orden de no resucitar fuera del hospital en la clínica ambulatoria si se presenta una copia de la directiva y el médico interviniente declara que coincide con la directiva. También tiene derecho a identificar a un tomador de decisiones sustituto para el caso en que usted se vea incapacitado mediante un Poder Médico.

Tomaremos sus dudas y reclamos con seriedad y trabajaremos duro para solucionarlos. Por lo tanto, estaremos atentos a sus necesidades y pedidos específicos, entendiendo que no deberían interferir con la atención médica para usted y los demás.

Usted tiene derecho a recibir una evaluación y el manejo oportuno y apropiado de su dolor. Le preguntaremos sistemáticamente si siente dolor. En caso afirmativo, lo evaluaremos y lo ayudaremos a obtener alivio.

Usted tiene derecho a que se respeten sus necesidades personales. Respetaremos la confidencialidad de su información personal en toda la institución y únicamente la divulgaremos de conformidad con las leyes y reglamentos aplicables. Para las personas en servicio activo, puede no ser posible mantener la confidencialidad completa, conforme a los requisitos de informar algunas condiciones y hallazgos. Respetaremos su necesidad de privacidad en las conversaciones, estudios, información compartida y procedimientos. Asimismo, puede solicitar la presencia de un acompañante durante un estudio o procedimiento. Tiene derecho a la divulgación total de la información sobre su salud y a la protección contra la divulgación no autorizada de la información sobre su salud.

Nos comunicaremos con usted en el idioma que pueda comprender. Podemos proporcionar intérpretes y servicios de traducción. Respetaremos su necesidad de sentirse seguro en todas las instalaciones. Los empleados del hospital serán identificados a través de distintivos o credenciales.

Usted tiene derecho a la seguridad física en nuestras instalaciones y nuestro personal de seguridad trabaja las 24 horas del día para garantizarle seguridad.

Usted tiene derecho a su dignidad y sus valores, creencias y preferencias religiosas, espirituales, culturales y psicosociales. Nuestros proveedores de atención pastoral y espiritual (a menudo llamados capellanes) llevan a cabo visitas diarias a los pacientes y se encuentran a su disposición.

Además, a pedido, coordinan otro apoyo espiritual que usted solicite siempre que no interfiera con su atención medica y la de otras pacientes o el funcionamiento del hospital.

Respetaremos su necesidad de comunicarse con otros, tanto familiares como amigos. Si es clínicamente necesario limitar su comunicación con otros, los mantendremos a usted y a su familia informados del motivo. Mientras esté internado, lo ayudaremos a realizar conversaciones telefónicas privadas, si lo desea.

Utilizaremos dispositivos de restricción física de tela suave con su monitoreo estricto y frecuente, si usted se encuentra en un estado de confusión tal que corra peligro de lastimarse a si misma o a otros. Quitaremos la restricción en cuanto podamos hacerlo con seguridad.

Usted tiene derecho a estar libre de abuso, negligencia y explotación en casa y en el hospital. Le haremos preguntas sobre estos temas para poder ayudarlo.

Usted tiene derecho a recibir información sobre como contactar servicios de protección. Si la solicita, le brindaremos información sobre como puede contactar servicios de protección y defensora para niños, adultos o ancianos.

Usted tiene derecho a participar en investigaciones clínicas cuando sea apropiado. Su proveedor de atención alanizara esto cuando sea apropiado. La Junta de Revisión Institucional, un comité que incluye a personas de muchas partes de esta comunidad, monitorea toda la investigación realizada en el BAMC. Le explicaremos detalladamente la investigación propuesta y solicitaremos su autorización escrita para participar. Si decide no participar en la investigación, esto no afectará la atención que le brindamos. La participación es completamente voluntaria.

Usted tiene derecho a hablar con un Representante de Pacientes de BAMC con respecto a cualquier aspecto de su atención, incluso para presentar una queja. Alentamos a los pacientes y sus familias a hablar directamente con el personal clínica o de guardia si hay un problema. No obstante, si estas personas no pueden resolverlo, puede comunicarse con el Representante de Pacientes al 210-916-2330 (clínica) o al 210-916-2200 (torre de pacientes internos).

Usted tiene derecho a esperar que esta institución funcione conforme a un código de comportamiento ético. Usted tiene derecho a estar involucrado en la resolución de dilemas con respecto a su atención, tratamiento y servicios. BAMC está firmemente comprometido a manejar este hospital conforme a las más elevadas tradiciones de profesionalismo y ética militares y médicas. Además, nuestro Comité de Bioética Institucional se reúne con regularidad para revisar temas éticos, incluyendo ética organizacional. Este comité está a su disposición y la de nuestros empleados si surge un dilema ético serio en la atención o los servicios de cualquier paciente.

Usted tiene derecho a recibir una copia personal de estos derechos de los pacientes. Las copias de estos derechos y responsabilidades de los pacientes están dispuestos en todas las guardias y clínicas de BAMC. Si no puede encontrar una copia, solicítela al personal de guardia o de clínicas.

Si tiene alguna pregunta o comentario con respecto a los derechos o responsabilidades de los pacientes, lo alentamos a que se comunique con un Representante de Pacientes de BAMC al 210-916-2330 (clínica) o al 210-916-2200 (torre de pacientes internos).

# Sus responsabilidades como paciente

Usted es responsable de maximizar sus propios comportamientos saludables.

Usted es responsable de brindarnos información precisa y completa sobre su salud y su estado.

Usted es responsable de tomar parte active en las decisiones sobre la atención de su salud. Usted es responsable de hacer preguntas y seguir las instrucciones de su médico.

Usted es responsable de mostrar cortesía y respeto hacia los otros pacientes, familiares, personal del hospital y visitas. Esto incluye el personal y los bienes del hospital.

Usted es responsable de ser puntual para sus citas programadas y de avisarnos con anticipación si debe cancelar o reprogramar una cita.

Usted es responsable de brindarnos su domicilio actual y los medios de contacto (tales como teléfono particular o celular).

Usted es responsable de brindarnos información actual sobre cualquier otra cobertura de seguro de salud que posea, y de asegurar que las obligaciones financieras asociadas con su atención se cumplan de manera oportuna.

# Appendix C-1

**XYZ Rehabilitation Clinic**
**654 First Avenue, SW**
**Majestic, USA 15551**
**(210) 555-HELP**

## Clinic Privacy Policy

**Effective date: April 16, 2003**

THIS NOTICE INFORMS YOU OF THE PROTECTIONS WE AFFORD TO YOUR PROTECTED HEALTH INFORMATION (PHI). PLEASE READ IT CAREFULLY.

**Purpose:** HIPAA, the Health Insurance Portability and Accountability Act of 1996, is a federal law addressing privacy and the protection of protected health information (PHI). This law gives you significant new rights as to how your PHI is used. HIPAA provides for penalties for misuse of PHI. As required by HIPAA, this notice explains how we are obliged to maintain the privacy of your PHI and how we are permitted, by law, to use and communicate it.

**Maintenance of records:** We utilize and communicate your PHI for the following reasons: treatment, reimbursement, and administrative medical operations.

- **Treatment** includes medical services delivered by professionals. Example: evaluation by a doctor or nurse.
- **Reimbursement** includes activities required for reimbursement for services, including confirming insurance coverage, sending bills and collection, and utilization review, among other things. Example: sending a bill for services to your company for payment.
- **Administrative medical operations** include the business of managing the clinic, including, improving the quality of services, conducting audits, and client services, among other things. Example: patient satisfaction surveys.

We also are permitted to create and distribute anonymous medical information by removing all references to PHI.

All of the employees of this clinic may see your records, as needed. We use sign-in and sign-out logs, containing the names of our patients in the waiting room, and we telephone patients to confirm appointments. We place your folder in a plastic in-box (with your name hidden) in the hallway in front of your treatment room.

When making photocopies of your records, we have your folder in our sight at all times, until we file it away with other folders. The medical records area is limited to employees only. When we send your PHI by fax, we ensure to the maximum extent possible that the receiving fax is secure.

All other uses of your PHI require your written authorization, including sharing your PHI with family members or others. You have the right to revoke any authorization in writing, and we have the legal duty to comply with such a revocation, except to the extent that we have used your information in reliance on your previous authorization, or as required by law.

**The right of patients to see, copy, and amend their medical records:** To take advantage of these rights, please present your request in writing to the clinic Privacy Officer (see below). You have the right to see your medical records. We will try to give you access as quickly as possible, depending on our workload. Within one week of your request, you may see your records in one of our offices, with the assistance of one of our employees. You have the right to make copies of your records. We have the right to charge for those copies. You may also request that the Privacy Officer honor special limitations on the uses and communications of your PHI. We are not obliged to comply with such requests. If we agree, we must comply with the request until you advise us in writing otherwise. You have the right to receive a copy of this notice, which we offer to you on your first visit. This notice, which is subject to change, is posted prominently in our waiting area.

**Privacy Officer:** The Privacy Officer for the clinic is _____, RN. Please speak with this employee about any question or complaint that you may have about your PHI. You may make special requests concerning your PHI.

**Correspondence with the patient:** We will send correspondence to the address that you have given us, but you have the right to ask that we send correspondence to a different address.

**Complaints:** If you feel that your PHI has not been treated with privacy, you may communicate this concern to the clinic Privacy Officer. You also have the right to communicate any problem to the Secretary of Health and Human Services (a division of the federal government) without being worried about retaliation by this clinic. We ask, though, that you first discuss and try to resolve any problem with our Privacy Officer. Thanks, and welcome to XYZ Clinic!

# Appendix C-2

**Clínica XYZ de Rehabilitación**
**654 First Avenue, SW**
**Majestic, USA 15551**
**(210) 555-HELP**

## Norma de Privacidad de la Clínica

**Effective date: April 16, 2003**

ESTA NOTICIA LE INFORMA SOBRE LAS PROTECCIONES
QUE TOMAMOS CON SU INFORMACIÓN MÉDICA PROTEGIDA.
HAGA EL FAVOR DE LEERLO CON CUIDADO.

**Intento:** HIPAA, el Health Insurance Portability and Accountability
Act of 1996, es una ley federal que trata con la privacidad y protección
de información médica protegida (IMP). Esta ley le da a usted, el
paciente, derechos significantes nuevos sobre como se utiliza su IMP.
HIPAA provee por penas por el mal uso de IMP.Como es requisito por
HIPAA, esta norma explica como estamos obligado de mantener la
privacidad de IMP y como estamos permitido usar y comunicar su IMP.

**Mantenimiento de los documentos:** Utilizamos y comunicamos su
IMP por las razones siguientes: el tratamiento, el pago y las operaciones
administrativas médicas.

- **Tratamiento** incluye servicios medicales entregados por profesionales. Ejemplo: evaluación por un médico o enfermera.
- **Pago** incluye actividades requisitos para el reembolso de servicios, incluyendo, entre otras cosas, confirmar los seguros, mandar facturas y coleccionar, y análisis de utilización.Ejemplo: mandar una factura a su compañía de seguro para pagar por servicios.
- **Operaciones administrativas médicas** incluyen el negocio de administrar la clínica, incluyendo, entre otras cosas, el mejoramiento de la calidad de servicios, hacer auditorias, y servicio de clientes.Ejemplo: encuestas de satisfacción.

También podemos hacer y distribuir información médica anónima por quitar todas referencias a la IMP.

Todos los empleados de esta clínica pueden ver sus documentos, si necesitan verlos. Usamos planillas de firmar al entrar y salir, anunciamos los nombres de nuestros pacientes en la sala de espera, y llamamos a pacientes para recordarles de sus citas.Pondremos su carpeta de documentos en un caja plástica (con nombre escondido) en el pasillo de su cuarto de tratamiento.

Al hacer copias de sus documentos, tendremos la carpeta en nuestra vista hasta que lo guardamos con las otras carpetas. La área en que guardamos las carpetas está limitada a sólo los empleados. Cuando mandamos sus documentos por fax, nos aseguramos lo más posible que el fax a donde lo mandamos está seguro.

Todos otros usos de su IMP requieren su autorización escrito, incluyendo el comportamiento de su IMP con familiares u otras personas. Tiene el derecho de revocar su autorización en escrito, y tenemos la responsabilidad de cumplir con tal revocación, excepto al punto que ya hemos usado la información dependiente de su autorización anterior, o cuando tenemos que comunicar información por ley.

**El derecho de los pacientes a ver, copiar y enmendar sus documentos médicos:** Para ejecutar estos derechos, por favor presente su petición en escrito al Oficial de la Privacidad (vea abajo). Usted tiene el derecho de ver sus documentos médicos. Trataremos de rápidamente darle acceso, dependiente en lo ocupado que estemos. Entre una semana después de su solicitud, podrá ver los documentos en una sala de esta oficina, con la asistencia de un empleado. Tendrá el derecho de hacer copias. Tenemos el derecho de cobrar por las copias. También puede pedir al Oficial de la Privacidad peticiones especiales sobre los usos y comunicaciones de su IMP. No tenemos que cumplir con estas peticiones. Si estamos de acuerdo, tenemos que seguir con la petición hasta que usted acuerde en escrito de quitarla. Tiene el derecho de tener una copia de esta noticia, que le ofrecemos en su primera visita a la clínica. Esta noticia, que se puede cambiar, está puesta prominentemente en la sala de recepción.

**Oficial de la Privacidad:** El Oficial de la Privacidad de la clínica es _____, RN. Por favor, hable con este empleado sobre cualquier pregunta o queja que tenga sobre su IMP. Puede pedirle cosas en especial sobre su IMP.

**Correspondencia al paciente:** Mandaremos cartas a la dirección que usted nos ha dado, pero tiene el derecho de pedir que las mandemos a otra dirección.

**Quejas:** Si usted piensa que su IMP no ha sido tratado con privacidad, usted puede comunicar este problema al Oficial de la Privacidad de la clínica. También tiene el derecho de comunicar cualquier problema al Secretario de *Health and Human Services* (una división del gobierno federal) sin preocupaciones de retaliación de esta clínica. Le rogamos que hable primeramente con el Oficial de la Privacidad para resolver sus problemas. Gracias y bienvenido a la clínica XYZ!

# Index

# W

# Notes

# Notes

# Notes

# Notes